Sisterhood of the Wounded Breast

Mary L. Maas

Copyright 2015 Mary L. Maas

ALL RIGHTS RESERVED. This book contains material protected under International and Federal Copyright Laws and Treaties. Any unauthorized reprint or use of this material is prohibited. No part of this book may be reproduced or transmitted in any form or by any means, electronic or mechanical, including photocopying, recording, or by any information storage and retrieval system without express written permission from the author/publisher.

Foreword

This book is a collection of memories from women who were willing to share their breast cancer experiences. Each of us wanted to tell about our journey through the doors leading into exam rooms, mammography machines, biopsy procedures, surgery, radiation and reconstruction. Each story is as unique as the individual who wrote it. Each story has been told in their own words in the hope of helping others who have recently been told they have breast cancer, as well as those who are traveling down the road to recovery.

Diagnostic procedures, treatments and follow-up tests have improved immensely through the years. The diagnosis of breast cancer no longer is an automatic death sentence. With all of the advancement in the breast cancer field, the diagnoses can be made at an earlier stage with the prognosis of a cure much more likely.

We have all suffered, in varying degrees, through biopsies, lumpectomies or mastectomies, radiation and some lingering side effects, due to lengthy recoveries or follow-up prescriptions.

The physical and mental strains needed to be handled with a positive attitude and determination to win.

We in the Breast Cancer Sisterhood want all of you who read our words to gain hope, encouragement and trust, in your doctor, your faith or your support groups.

I want to thank all the contributors to this book and I appreciate their candor. Not all the steps through their journeys were easy. But it is our hope that reading about those who have conquered the battle and are victorious will give others a positive attitude towards reaching the same goal.

The book is dedicated to all those who met Cancer head on and fought the valiant fight to win.

It is also dedicated in memory of Carol S. Campbell who fought the good fight.

Mary L. Maas

Contents

Chapter One – Rita M. Roenfeldt 1

Chapter Two – Deb Maas 4

Chapter Three – Jean Sherlock 16

Chapter Four – Alice Herbolsheimer 41

Chapter Five – Elaine Roessle 43

Chapter Six – Barbara J. (Boyd) Wolverton 48

Chapter Seven – Jo Mandl 54

Chapter Eight – Terry Warnke 61

Chapter Nine – Charlie 68

Chapter Ten – Agnes Jeanette Hoagland 78

Chapter Eleven – Shelly Bentz 85

Chapter Twelve – Lora Johnson 91

Chapter Thirteen – Claudie Wilson 99

Chapter Fourteen – Pam 105

Chapter Fifteen – Beverly C. 150

Chapter Sixteen – Carole S. Campbell, Ph.D.. . . . 155

Chapter Seventeen – Linda S. 159

Chapter Eighteen – Suzy 166

Chapter Nineteen – Patricia A. Howard 169

Chapter Twenty – Deb 174

Chapter Twenty-One – Rita Robinson Brown. . . 177

Chapter Twenty-Two – Janice/AKA: OZ. 187

Chapter Twenty-Three – Mary L. Maas 218

CHAPTER ONE

RITA M. ROENFELDT

For the past 30-plus years, three of my friends and I have traveled to Omaha, NE., (110 miles one way) to have our annual physicals and mammograms with an OB/GYN physician. Every year, when each of us comes out after our appointment, we all wonder how they have fared with the doctor.

Well, 2012 was the first time that any one of us received a majorly negative report and it happened to be me. My doctor found a lump in my left breast about the size of a small olive. I always had the feeling that I would, more than likely, have breast cancer. My mother had a breast removed when she was 65 years old and my youngest sister had recently died from lung and brain cancer at age 56.

I was very thankful that my friends were there for me. They kept my mind busy with other things, so I didn't dwell on it. I returned to Omaha the following week for a biopsy. Later that week, I received a call from my surgeon that it was breast cancer.

I returned to Omaha again for an MRI and the next week I met with an oncologist. I thought she was going to tell me what they were going to do and when. Instead, she gave me the options for which decisions I needed to make. Did I want a lumpectomy or a total breast removed? This was a hard decision for me and I went to two of my church family members who had gone through breast cancer previously. They told me their experiences and the reason for the treatment(s) they chose. It was still hard for me to decide, but since the lump was small, I decided to have a lumpectomy.

The surgeon told me he thought I'd made the right choice and that radiation would follow surgery. But when the lab report came back after surgery, they had found two small flecks, the size of a sharp pencil tip, in my lymph glands.

I received four chemotherapy treatments. I had quite a battle with keeping my white blood cell count up. After my second chemo treatment, the oncologist told me I had no white blood cells at all. This meant I could not be around people. I could not eat fresh fruits or vegetables. I went to the CDU unit at the hospital for a neupogen shot three or four times a week. This shot stimulates the bone marrow to produce white blood cells.

After my fourth chemo treatment, I had six weeks, five days a week, of radiation treatments. These treatments went well. It took longer to get undressed and dressed than it did for the actual treatment. I was thankful I was able to have all my treatments in Norfolk, a nearby city about 12 miles away. I finished the treatments the week before Christmas. What a Christmas present!

In May 2013, I had my first follow-up mammogram, chest x-ray, and blood work done. Everything came out good, so now I don't have to go back until September, except to have my port flushed monthly.

I pray every day that I won't have a recurrence.

Chapter Two

Deb Maas

I grew up the youngest of seven children, five girls and two boys. We lived on a farm and were always a close and supportive family. I was born and raised Catholic and faith was a big part of my upbringing. I have always believed that God had a plan for everyone and cancer was part of his plan for me.

The journey:
02-05: I found the lump
02-09: ultrasound
02-10: mammogram/ultrasound

I believe this ultrasound was checking the lymph nodes as well as the lump and surrounding area.

02-17: biopsy in Albion

What I remember being the worst at this time was the waiting. Go to an appointment, wait a week. Days would drag on and no phone calls with results.

When the results of the biopsy finally came back they called me on my cell phone when I was at work and the only thing that I totally remember is them saying "the type of cancer you have is…" The rest of the conversation was kind of a blur. All I knew at that point was that I had cancer.

I met my husband, Derric, at our house, and all we could do was cry. We didn't know much about the type or treatment or anything. So more appointments were made and then there was more waiting.

02-25: MRI/Albion

I had no experience with an MRI, and that particular day, I was sick with a head cold and laying face down on a table for the MRI was no fun at all. I was nervous and I had no idea what they would find and I was praying for the best.

03-04 Dr. B.

Once again, the waiting was terrible. If you look at the dates between appointments, they are not that far apart, but at the time, it seemed like forever. I wanted to get the results, have "it" removed and get back to normal life.

Dr. B. informed us that it was a lump about the size of a dime, but the MRI also showed a small spot about an inch from the lump that they wanted to check. So another ultrasound was scheduled to see if the small spot could be found with an ultrasound and not just on the MRI.

03-09 ultrasound

The small spot was detected on the ultrasound.

03-11: Dr. B.

Consulting with Dr. B., he gave the options available to me. My first thought would be mastectomy and no chemo. It was all my choice, but Dr. B. is more conservative and suggested lumpectomy and radiation. We could always go more "drastic" if or when necessary. I would have the lumpectomy, have removal of the smaller spot next to it, have it all tested and go from there.

03-16: Surgery

Surgery was out patient and pretty uneventful. I was home by that afternoon and returned to work the next day. My entire mindset was to have the treatments that I needed, take care of the family, work and get it all over ASAP.

03-21: mammogram/ultrasound

This appointment seemed to have arrived quicker than I had wanted for the first time since February. I was not sure how I could possibly have a mammogram this quickly after surgery. Well, I did have it and all was good. There was no sign of any lump or spot.

At some point throughout the visits, I took what they called an Oncotype DX test to see my recurrence risk. I decided to have this test thinking this would be the perfect way to reassure myself that chemotherapy would not be necessary. I had a follow-up on the test with Dr. M.

03-24: Dr. M.

This appointment was a great disappointment in the results. My results showed that chemo was recommended. I still did not want to HAVE to have it, but this again was my decision. I'd said from the beginning that I would trust in what the doctors said and recommended, and I would do whatever was necessary to get through this with no regrets.

04-22: first chemo

This is a day you never want to see come. Walking into the chemo room and looking around at the other patients sitting around, hooked up to the drug that was to help them was pretty scary. It was obvious to me that there were some pretty sick people in that room and I was not nearly as bad off as I could have been. Still the thought of sitting down and dripping that into your system is a pretty shocking situation. Just to know that is what you need but not at all what you want and of course, I knew the loss of my hair was soon to come. You would like that it should be no big deal in the scope of things, but it was a big deal.

Dr. M. said that not all people lose their hair, but most do. I did get my hair cut quite short, as my hair was always fairly long, but at no point was I able to shave it off. In 14 to 21 days was the time frame they gave for the significant hair loss to begin and that was pretty true to form for me.

While sitting at work one day, I remember just reaching up and pulling on a small amount of my hair just to see if, in fact, it was coming out like they had said, and sure enough it was. I really didn't need to do this for reassurance, because if I simply looked at my clothes and shower floor, as well as when I blew dry my hair, it was obvious that it was falling out.

After several more thousand tears and sleepless nights, and of course cleaning up a lot of hair, I eventually began to wear a wig.

05-13: second chemo

I did not have a shunt put in and just received my chemo through a regular IV. It was strange to me how you could feel the IV through your veins. They told me I was actually feeling the "rinse" between the drugs and it was because it was a different temperature than the chemo drugs. I have not had much experience with IVs and hospitals or with any treatment in general, so I didn't know much. Two of my friends insisted on going to the treatments with me and sat there and did their best to keep the four to five hours of treatment as light as they could be. As they were sitting there, chatting away on one particular session, I began to feel really hot, I felt my face turn hot and my ears were burning up. As I interrupted my friends conversation, they looked at me and panicked a bit! I was bright red and was having an allegic reaction to my treatment. They called the nurse over who shut down the treatment. They did a flush and gave me the treatment at a slower pace and all was well. They asked me if I had taken the prescription that was given to me to take before each treatment. I said …no… did I have a prescription? And was I supposed to take something before treatments? I guess that was one of the things that got by me in my previous appointment. I have to admit that there were many times that I simply stopped listening, because I probably did not want to hear what they were saying. It was hard to focus on the situation at hand and I am sure taking notes would probably have been a good option for me.

06-02: third chemo

As the treatments went on they continued to take a bit more out of me each time. I would go to a treatment on Wednesday, go to work on Thursday and Friday "like normal". Thursday was good, but by Friday afternoon the treatment would start to bring me down. I went home from work on Friday and had very limited energy for Saturday and Sunday. I went back to work on Monday through Friday of the next week. Just when I would start to feel pretty well, it was back to treatment.

06-24: fourth chemo

I don't remember anything extra "special" about the last treatment. My friends, my sister and my husband continued to be there throughout it all. I had asked the boys if they wanted to come or even to see the treatment room and they didn't want anything to do with it. That was fine with me. I can be quite sure that after I finished my treatments, the chemo room must have seemed rather quiet, because I was never alone, not one time and we were not a quiet group either.

Radiation:

This was really pretty uneventful. The set up took a bit but once all was set, things rolled right along. Thank goodness, I was able to do the radiation treatments in Norfolk, NE. I would go in at 8 a.m. and be out in 15 to 20 minutes. It took longer for me to change clothes than it did for the treatment. I had a couple delays for machine maintenances, but this treatment went pretty smooth. When I start the first of 40 sessions, I thought it would never end. I continued to work every day, run after the boys and attend their sports every evening. I was more tired than I expected, but they said that was due to coming off chemo and going right into radiation. I have some skin discoloration from the treatments and of course the "tattooed" markings are all that remain after the entire process.

After all the treatments were completed, we had a party and my family gave me a very nice ring for the celebration. It is a constant reminder that all I went through was worth it and their support was with me all the way.

I continued to wear my wig until mid December and finally I got brave enough to go out with my new,

VERY short and VERY curly hair. The curl did not stay with me and eventually my normal hair returned.

The report:

TNM staging: TIC Pathologic N, PNO, MO, Location: left breast

Histology: Invasive ductal carcinoma. Histologic grade: 2. Lymphovascular invasion: nine. ER/PR: ER status: positive, PR statue: positive. HER-2/neu: Receptor status: IHC overexpression O. Ki-67/MIB-I: LI: High

Oncotype DX, recurrence score: RS: 32, 10 year risk for recurrence: high risk (rs=> 31)

Completed treatment details:

Surgery – Lumpectomy with sentinel lymph node biopsy (h/o) 03-16-09, left.

Chemotherapy – Docetaxel +cyclophosphamide (tc) (h/o): Start date 04-22-09. Finish date 06-24-09. Number of cycles: 4.

Radiotherapy – External beam radiation to primary tumor site (h/o): Start date: 07-23-09, Finish date: 09-11-09.

Hormone Therapy: Tamoxifen (h/o): Start 09-16-09. Change to Aromasin 03-21-2012

Current status: no evidence of disease.

#

My husband and two boys were a very important part of what I went through with my cancer. When I first found the lump, I told only my husband and my sister who lived in the same town as we do. I didn't want to "alarm" anyone, especially the boys, if there was no reason for concern. It was not until after my biopsy and results that we sat down with the boys to give them the news. The oldest was age 16, a sophomore in high school, and the youngest age 13, a 7th grader. Our house was always the hangout for their friends, so I just asked the boys to try to avoid having friends over and as soon as we got through this, all could be back to normal. As a sophomore, our oldest knew what was happening, but did his best to avoid any conversation about it and so we just didn't talk much about it unless we had to. At age thirteen, our youngest was okay to just play video games and not worry about what we were dealing with. I found it easier to let him play his video games, than to ask how he felt about what was going on.

My husband's cousin, who had lost her mom to cancer at a similar age, was one of the first to be told and she was a good source of security for the boys. She was very honest with them, as we were, but they knew they could go to her anytime they felt they might need to. We all shared a lot of tears.

The boys continued school and their sports activities through it all. We all went about our busy lives as though nothing had changed, but every day was still different. I knew everyone knew what I was going through, but we all just kind of kept our distance. I had a hard time talking about any of it and I really didn't know what to say or "how to be". I didn't know how to be the mom with cancer; all I really wanted to do was to make it as easy as possible for the boys. We just didn't talk about it much.

Whenever I had a chemo treatment, I would ask them if they were interested in coming with or if they wanted to see the treatment room. Their answers were always, NO! They were good! I didn't blame them for wanting to ignore the situation; that was all I wanted to do, too, but knew we had to face it head on.

I had all the support in the world from family and friends. I received cards and flowers throughout the process, along with prayer after prayer. Never underestimate the power of prayer. It has taken me quite some time to open up and actually talk about cancer. Part of me just wants to put it in the past, and talking about it just brings it all right back to my mind. I have attended our Relay for Life every year since I have been a survivor, and yet I have not been able to participate in that first survivor lap! It is still just a little too much. I am not sure why. Maybe someday I will walk that first lap, but for now, I will just stand back and count my blessings as the other survivors walk. I have become brave enough to actually wear the purple shirt, so time does heal. I am extremely thankful for being a survivor, but I am also a very emotional person, so I prefer to stand back and cry in the midst of the crowd, at least for now.

There were a zillion tears I shed by myself and I am sure by my husband as well. He gave me space knowing full well that if I wanted to talk about anything that was going on, I would let him know. I can be sure that his side of the ordeal was not much easier than my own. We all made it through with a lot of love, support and understanding. Don't get me wrong, it was a tough, long haul, but we did it and we did it as a family.

Looking back I have to say that from the medical stand point, I thought it could have been a lot worse. I was never really sick, just extremely tired, overwhelmed and ached like I had shin splints in my entire body. My lumpectomy did not make a huge change to my body, so that was never a concern for me. The follow-up visits were really hard at first, I would panic thinking about the appointment coming up and then I would stress and worry until I got the results of each follow-up. They do get easier with time, but there is still always the worry and the concern of results that may not be what we want. For me, the mental part was worse than the medical. I am a pretty matter-of-fact person and I truly believe that what got me through was, first, the support of all my family and friends, and second, a positive attitude. I said from the start that I would do what had to be done, get it over with as soon as possible and I refused to let it get me down.

I realize that everyone has a different journey and everyone approaches things differently, but I believe that God, family and friends can get anyone through anything.

My five years is here since my cancer journey and sometimes it feels like forever ago and yet, at other times, it feels like it was yesterday. Our oldest is now a junior in college and our youngest is just about to graduate high school. Where has the time gone?

The bumps, along our paths of life, have made us all stronger, and they have made us the persons and family that we are today.

Stay strong, be positive and have faith that all will work out. Not a day goes by that I don't think about being a cancer survivor and I thank God for what he has given me…my family and my friends.

Chapter Three

Jean Sherlock

Breast cancer is a diagnosis that all women fear hearing from their doctor. It was during the spring of 2005 when I went in for my mammogram that changed my life forever. I was 42 years old and a single parent of two young girls, ages 12 and 9.

I really didn't have any symptoms that would lead me to even think I might have breast cancer, but I felt as if something just wasn't right. There were no lumps, swelling, redness or discharge from my nipple. I had two perfectly healthy looking breasts. I made an appointment to see my gynecologist and she did an examination. Not finding anything, she was quite happy to report a clean bill of health. Not feeling comfortable with this, I asked for a mammogram and she obliged with no questions or arguments. A couple of days after my mammogram, I received a call from the radiology department at Kaiser asking me to go in for a magnification mammogram since there was an area that needed further evaluation. Ninety five percent of these turn out to be nothing, I was told, but anything that looks a little suspicious is evaluated further. I went in the next day and had the magnification mammogram. Curious that I am, I asked the technician if I could see the image on the screen to see what they were looking at. The area was pointed out to me and I was sent on my way, after being reassured by the technician that 95% of these tests are normal and I really shouldn't worry. I was told that I would receive a call within a couple of days from the radiologist with the results.

A couple of days went by, and then a week, and then two weeks and still no word. This is normally a good sign "no news is good news". I placed a call to the radiology department and they were surprised that I had not been called. Within a few hours I received a call from a very nice radiologist letting me know that upon further evaluation she felt that a biopsy was warranted since I had micro-calcifications in three different areas on my left breast. However, she said not to worry because ninety five percent of micro-calcifications turn out to be benign. This is 95% of the 5% so the chance of my results coming back abnormal is very slim. Of course, although we try not to worry, since after all, there is only a slight chance that I might have cancer; it is very hard to not worry and start thinking about all of the possible scenarios.

After hanging up with the radiologist, I immediately went to the computer and started looking up images of micro-calcifications. In my head, I could see quite clearly the image from my mammogram. I found several that looked exactly like mine and it was then that I realized that I had breast cancer (unofficially). A very good friend of mine had breast cancer about seven years prior so I asked her to go with me when I was having my biopsy, which she happily agreed to. Having her there for me was very comforting.

Well, the day of the biopsy arrived (Tuesday) and off I went off to Kaiser, with my friend. The table where you lie for the needle core biopsy allows your breast to fall through holes. Not the most comfortable or flattering position to be in. In addition to the radiologist and nurse, the representative of the needle core biopsy machine was also present. The breast is numbed, placed into a mammogram machine and the needle inserted for the biopsy. Not really painful, just a little uncomfortable. My biopsy took about two and half hours to complete because one of the areas that showed on the initial mammogram could not be found for some reason. Good news, I thought. Maybe it is no longer there.

The biopsy was done without incident. I had three little metal markers left in my breast to identify the area where the suspicious micro-calcifications had been removed. Again, curiosity got the better of me and I asked if I could see the samples that had been taken from my breast. There were lots of stringy looking pink tissues lying on the tray, so many I was convinced my breast would look concave in the three areas the biopsies had been taken from. Odd to think that all that tissue had just been pulled from my breast. My breast was dressed with gauze and tape and I went home to wait. I was told that I could call the breast cancer nurse on Friday, after 12 noon for the results. Three days of waiting. Normally this is not a long time but in a situation like this, three days can feel like an eternity.

After the biopsy, one thing the nurses tell you is not to take any form of aspirin for at least 7 days because it thins your blood and causes bleeding. I developed a really bad headache and I needed something for pain so I took Excedrin without thinking. This was not a good idea. The bruising on my breast got a lot worse and my breast was black and blue for weeks.

12:05 on Friday I called the breast cancer nurse and was told that my results were in and that unfortunately, I had breast cancer. I was driving down Ygnacio Valley Road in Walnut Creek, CA at the time so I pulled over into a parking lot and called my friend to give her the news. For some odd reason, I was not surprised and took the news quite well. I was on my way to her house anyway to go walking but Kaiser had said that I could see them at 2:00pm to go over the results and I wanted my friend to go with me. My friend Nancy was quite surprised to hear the news but was so organized and on top of everything. When I got to her house she already had note pads out and had started writing down questions that we needed to ask the nurse.

As soon as we got to Kaiser we were taken in to the nurse's office. As she was explaining everything to me, Nancy was writing everything down because she knew that later I would probably not remember everything. Boy, was she right. The confirmative diagnosis of breast cancer still had not really sunk it. Yes, I knew I had cancer, but what did it really mean? How was this going to affect my family and me? The nurse was very sweet and understanding and kept asking if I had any questions. I would look down at my note pad and see if anything applied to what we were talking about. It was too soon to know at what stage I was and this would not be known until after I had had my surgery.

I had cancer in three different locations on the breast, 9 o'clock, 12 o'clock and 3 o'clock so I was informed that a lumpectomy was probably not an option for me. I would almost for sure need the mastectomy, however, the surgeon would confirm this when I saw him on Monday. A friend had loaned me a book called "Reconstructing Aphrodite" which was about women who had breast reconstruction after a mastectomy. It was full of women of all ages who had gone through breast cancer. Seeing this makes you realize that you are not alone is this venture and hundreds of women before me had trodden this path. I already knew from talking with Nancy that I would want the tran flap re-construction so the nurse had us watch the video that Kaiser required you to watch if you were considering that procedure. It was very informative and I felt totally comfortable with my decision. As I was watching the movie though, the faces of my two little girls kept popping into my mind. Am I going to be around to watch them grow up, graduate high school, go to college and get married.

As we left Kaiser, the main thoughts going through my mind was "what do I tell my girls?" Should I even tell them? Of course, I knew that the right thing was to tell them the truth. As I was driving over to school to pick them up, I called my ex-husband (We are best friends) and gave him the news. He was shocked and couldn't really say much except that he would be there for me. I picked the girls up from school and went to Nancy's house for dinner and wine, a much-needed glass of wine.

My daughters had very different personalities so I decided to tell them separately. Jillian, my youngest, spent the night with her friend Mackenzie, Nancy's daughter, and Sarah and I went home. In the car I had Sarah's undivided attention so I took the opportunity to tell her. She listened while looking at me in horror and when I had finished talking she asked me two questions; Mom, are you going to die? And can she get it? It broke my heart to hear her ask these questions. I held her hand as I explained to her that I didn't have all of the information yet from the doctor, but from what the nurse told me, I was pretty sure that I was going to be OK. We had caught my cancer early. As far as whether or not she could get it, that was a tough one. So, my answer was that anyone can get cancer, it doesn't matter who you are, but so long as you take care of your body, get regular checkups and if you feel like anything is wrong with your body, have the doctor take a look, and then you should be ok. I didn't know what else to say. I knew what my daughter was thinking. My mother and father both died from cancer so in her little mind, if you got cancer, you died. Lots of hugs and snuggles were in order for that night.

The next day I picked Jillie up from Nancy's and again on the way home, I explained to her what was going on. She looked at me and said "ok mom I get it. I don't want to hear any more". That was it. Now of course, she was only 9 and didn't really understand what cancer was, except that it can kill you. She wouldn't hug me, kiss me, touch me or even come close to me for several weeks. Although I understood, I still felt a little hurt that my baby wouldn't even give me a hug. In the meantime I decided to take both girls to a therapist for a few visits because they had a hard time talking to me about their feelings. They didn't want to hurt me or to even really see them cry. I did find out from the therapist though that Jillian had thought that she could get cancer by touching me so once it was explained to her that she couldn't catch it, she slowly started coming around.

Now the slew of appointments and waiting began. I had appointments with the general surgeon, plastic surgeon, oncologist, bone scan, PET scan. My Auntie Beat and Uncle George came over from England to be with me for a few months to help out in any way they could. They also provided emotional support for me and just listened when I needed to talk. I couldn't have made it through my cancer without their help. My mother and father had both passed away, so they could not be there for me. Auntie Beat, my mother's sister, has become like a mother to me and George like a father. They mean the world to me.

Nancy went with me to see the general surgeon, who explained as we thought, that a lumpectomy was not an option. The cancer was in three different spots and invasive, so I needed to have a mastectomy. This did not come as too much of a shock to me as the nurse had already mentioned this is probably the procedure I would need. For my own piece of mind, I discussed having a bilateral mastectomy but the physician talked me out of it stating the chances of getting breast cancer on the other side are very slim. I went along with his plan, however every day I have regretted not pushing for the bi-lateral mastectomy. We are the ones who worry every time we have to go in for a mammogram, especially if we are called back again for a magnification. Having the bilateral mastectomy would have eliminated this future worry. If I was 21 and looking for a spouse, I might think differently about having a mastectomy, but I was 42 and my breasts were not that important to me. I would much rather have peace of mind.

The plastic surgeon appointment was next. I walked in to the office and was taken to an examining room by the nurse. On my way back, we walked by a physician's office where a youngish man with long blonde hair was sitting at his computer. I am not a fan of men with long hair and I prayed to God he was not my physician. A few minutes later there was a knock at the door and THAT physician walked in. My heart sank. The doctor introduced himself and gave a big beaming smile and instantly I felt at ease. How could I be so judgmental? He spent so much time talking with me and explaining the procedure, and constantly displaying his heart-warming smile and by the time I left the office I was so glad he was my physician. Within an hour I had completely changed my opinion on this one physician. I could not have been more wrong about someone.

My oncologist informed me I would need to have chemotherapy after the surgery. The thought of having chemotherapy made me turn sick. Having cancer and a mastectomy was nowhere near as horrifying as having chemo. After my appointment with the oncologist, I had an appointment with the pharmacist and then a tour of the chemo unit. Thank heaven I had my Auntie Beat with me otherwise I don't think I would have made it. We walked into the unit and there were pods with about 8-10 chairs in each pod. Every chair was full. Some people were sitting there chatting with family members as if nothing was out of the norm; others were sitting there staring into space and some were moaning as if in terrible pain. I felt horrified and it was all I could do to hold my tears back. I didn't want chemo; I didn't want to be like any of these people; I didn't want to lose my hair; I wanted my "normal" life back. Whose nightmare was I in? We left the unit and drove home in silence. I could not say a word.

Reality hit and I knew I was going to lose my hair. Rather than wait for that time to arrive, I decided now was a good time to find a wig; one that looked similar to my hair. The cancer unit at Kaiser had told me the American Cancer Society has a lot of free items people with cancer can have for free, including wigs. I went there and tried on several wigs finally picking out one that I liked but was not really similar to my current natural hair. I then went and bought another wig from the wig shop so I could have a change. Wigs are not cheap and being the frugal shopper that I am, I naturally had to find one on sale. The average cost of a wig was $130 and I was so happy that I was able to buy one for $30. Shampoo, conditioner, scalp net and head for the wigs came to about another $40 so I walked out of the door for around $70. The cost of a haircut I thought so this made me feel better.

The time leading up to the surgery seemed to last forever. I decided this time was valuable and I should enjoy it as much as possible. I had a strange feeling something was going to happen during my surgery and that I may not make it. This was a feeling I couldn't share with anyone, but I was getting very nervous, as the time of the surgery got closer. I got all of my affairs in order; made a will and living trust, completed my health care initiative and gave a copy to Kaiser, my auntie and uncle and my ex-husband, wrote a list of the life insurance policies I had and where the information could be found and I wrote letters to both of my girls. I didn't want to exit this world and not have them know just how much I love them. I felt prepared and comfortable when the day of my surgery arrived.

Tuesday, June 7, 2005 finally arrived and off I went to the hospital at 7am, with Auntie Beat and

Sisterhood of the Wounded Breast

George in tow. It was going to be a long day for everyone. I was checked in and taken to the pre-op area. Auntie Beat stayed with me the whole time while the nurses got me ready and finally my doctors came in to do a final examination prior to surgery. First the general surgeon came in and then the plastic surgeon. I felt like an art board as the plastic surgeon drew on my breast and stomach in permanent marker. He was marking the area for the general surgeon to cut on the breast, making sure the area was the right size to save enough skin for the tran flap reconstruction. The area on my stomach was huge and I looked at the amount of skin in the middle and wondered how on earth I would be able to stand straight with that much skin removed. My belly button would be cut out and sewn back into the new area. Oh boy. I had also asked for a porta cath to be inserted for the chemo so I would not have to have it through the veins in my arms. This was a relatively easy procedure and only added 20 minutes to the general surgeon's time.

Out in the waiting room my family was advised to go home and relax as the surgery was going to take 9-10 hours. Auntie Beat and George went home to anxiously wait for the call advising them I was out of surgery and in recovery. 6:30 pm they received the call and was told they could visit me in a couple of hours.

Mary L. Maas

I remember the plastic surgeon talking to me in the recovery room and telling me it is time to wake up. The very first words out of my mouth were "I am alive". I was so thankful to have made it through the surgery and know that my biggest fear of dying had not come to reality. I was alive! One of the nurses came and informed me that my ex-husband was here and would like to come in and see me. They seemed shocked when I said that is fine and assured them we were very good friends. It was not too long before I was wheeled up to my room to be greeted by my auntie and uncle. They were such troopers. After being under anesthesia for almost 10 hours, I could barely stay awake and I am sure they sat in the room and stared at me for a couple of hours before leaving for the night.

When I awoke the next morning, Auntie Beat and George were sitting in the exact same seats, staring at me just as they had done the night before. I remember asking them if they had been there all evening. It was still extremely difficult for me to stay awake so I nodded on and off throughout the day. On the wall behind my bed was a huge sign warning the nurses to not lay my bed down flat and to keep it in a semi reclined position. Within a day, the nurses had me out of bed walking up and down the corridors with a walker. I felt like I was standing at a 45 degree angle, and I probably was not too far off. A significant amount of skin had been cut from my stomach in order to do the Tran flap reconstruction and it was like I had had a tummy tuck. There were two drains coming out of my stomach, one on each side and one drain coming out of my breast. These were uncomfortable as they were stitched in place and sometimes movement would cause them to get caught or pulled.

My stay in the hospital was supposed to be 7-10 days but on Thursday evening (after only 2 days) my doctor informed me that I was doing so well he was going to discharge me on Friday and send me home. I could feel panic setting in. Go home, so soon? I hadn't even had a bowel movement. I was not on solid food or liquids yet so how could I be going home. My doctor said I will be more comfortable at home and there is less chance of getting an infection. Of course I was happy to be going home to sleep in my own bed, sit on the couch and relax but I was scared. Auntie Beat and George would do everything they could to make sure I was comfortable and taken care of, but what if something happened? What if I fell?

As planned, I was discharged home early Friday afternoon, stocked with pain pills and supplies for emptying my drains, which would stay in for another week or so. Auntie Beat and George always called me Angel so they had made a halo and put it over my headboard for me. I felt like an angel and could not have had any better of a welcome home gift. My two daughters were staying with friends for a couple more days so I could get settled in and not be too much of a burden on Auntie Beat and George. It was nice to be home but a little challenging. I couldn't sit on the sofa as it was too low so I had to put several cushions down first. I was still unable to lie flat and trying to stay in a seated position in bed all night also posed as a challenge, even with cushions under my legs. Every time I needed to get out of bed or move, I needed help and going downstairs was not the easiest of tasks. However, I never let any of this stop me from trying to get better and try to do things for myself.

One way I was able to find some relaxation was by taking a bath. I could only have about six inches of water in the bathtub due to the drains coming out of my stomach, but lying in the water was soothing. My auntie shaved my legs and underarms for me instantly making me feel like a new woman. Washing my hair could not be done in the bath tub as the water would travel down my back and front and could get into the areas where the drains were protruding from the skin so this was done in the kitchen sink, with me leaning forward. I was not complaining at all though as it felt really nice to be clean and after all, I was alive!

A few days passed and a rash started to develop around one of the drain sites on my stomach. We had been so careful to keep the area clean, used gloves when emptying the drains and sterilized everything around the house. A visit to the doctor was warranted and the diagnosis was a staph infection, requiring a shot of strong antibiotic in my bottom. This will do the trick the doctor said and he was right. Within a few days the infection had gone.

During this whole time the anesthesia had still not completely left my body and from time to time I would act a little crazy. I didn't realize it at the time but people later told me how they had never seen me act that way before. It is amazing how long the anesthesia stays in your body. I can see now why they say never to make important decisions soon after surgery.

My ten-day post surgical appointment arrived and I was placed in the examining room with my auntie. The examining room was not very big. The nurse came in to take off the dressings and then the on-call plastic surgeon, followed by the general surgeon and the physician assistant. I was amazed to see all of these people in one room, chatting and waiting to see the results of the reconstruction. Everyone seemed very pleased with how it looked. There was only one little problem; my belly button did not survive the transplant. It had "died" and was all black and nasty. Unfortunately, nothing could be done about this and I would no longer have a belly button. The thought of this was kind of funny, as I didn't know anyone who didn't have a belly button.

The plastic surgeon did say I would have a scar there and eventually it would look a little like a belly button. He wasn't lying.

The drains were finally taken out and I was told I could take a shower. That was like music to my ears. I had missed taking showers. Sitting in a bath with 3" of water and washing my hair in the kitchen sink was not quite the same. I couldn't wait to get home. Before I left the doctor's office, I was told my chemo would start the first week of July, which was only one week away. My excitement about going home and taking a shower was now subdued with the thought of beginning chemo in one week. Why so soon? Could it not wait? I need time to recover from the surgery. I tried to come up with as many excuses as I could as why I should wait a little while before starting the chemo, however, the reasons presented to me by my medical team were much more convincing so the date was set for my first chemo. I scheduled a Friday so I would have the weekend to recoup before having to do things with the girls. And, it gave me a few more days in between now and the start. At least I had the porta cath and would not have to endure the chemo going through my arms, which I had heard was not very pleasant. The porta cath, about the size of a stack of five quarters, was noticeable under my skin an inch or so below my right collarbone. It was hard to not keep playing with it.

That first shower when I arrived home was wonderful. I think I stayed in there for twenty to thirty minutes. I don't remember ever enjoying a shower so much and feeling so clean. I had to wear a special bra and girdle for three more weeks, but at least I could take those off while showering. These were tight garments to help from putting stress on the incisions and to help reduce bleeding. Although they weren't the most comfortable items to wear, they were not too bad and certainly bearable. I had a little over a week to shop, relax and prepare for the unknown. I had no idea how I was going to feel, if I would be able to eat, if I would be sick. I felt like I had no idea what was happening in my life. Just a few months earlier I was going about my business without a care in the world and now my life had been turned upside down. Nothing seemed normal any more. Even my girls looked at me differently and were afraid to come near me, just in case they caught the "cancer". Trying to convince them it is not contagious was not easy and it was hard for me to not let my feelings feel hurt. They were just kids and they would come around eventually. They would want to hug and kiss me again, this I knew.

The dreadful day arrived and off my auntie and I went to my first chemo session. Thank God I had my Auntie Beat with me. Without her, I don't know how I would have got through all of this. My mother had died from leukemia in 1997 and my dad from colon cancer in 2002. Auntie Beat and George dropped everything and came to help me get through this. Sitting in the seat waiting for my chemo, I was looking around the room at all the other people wondering what type of cancer they had. This seemed to be the popular hangout for people of all ages. As soon as one person vacated his or her seat, someone came in and filled it. The nurse came over and verified who I was and what I was there for. She explained the process and what drugs I would be given, then promptly inserted the needle into my porta cath. The drugs began to drip. This horrible poison was entering my body, but for a good cause. This poison was going to kill any cancer cell that may have come loose and travelled to other parts of my body. This poison was going to save me.

Well, I was pleased the process was not too painful at all. In fact, I didn't feel anything and felt wonderful when I left. We went home and I felt like eating a curry, so Auntie Beat and George made the best curry in the world. I devoured it. My auntie and I went shopping after dinner and this was when it all hit me. I started to feel strange, couldn't stand still and knew I needed to get home. I walked in the house and stripped off my clothes. I couldn't stand anything touching my skin and my brain felt like it was full of worms eating it. Rolling around on the floor like a crazy person was what my girls saw when they walked in. Wonderful, now they are really not going to want to come near me. My auntie called Kaiser to let them know what was going on and they went over all of my medications. I was missing two very important ones, which they had forgotten to give me. They called my ex-husband who drove over 20 miles to get the prescriptions for me. Not long after I took them I started to feel much better. How could they have forgotten to give me two important medications? This should be second nature to the nurses and doctors to make sure patients have everything.

The next day I started the vomiting and could not stop. Anti-nausea medications were prescribed to take before chemo, which I took, however, for some reason they were not working. I was admitted to the hospital for a couple of days for re-hydration. The doctor said some people still have this reaction, even with the anti-nausea meds so the day before my next chemo I was to go to the hospital and receive hydration. This made the world of difference. Even though the chemo makes your brain feel funny, there was no more nausea and vomiting. I just felt like I had drunk a bottle of whiskey.

Not everyone loses his or her hair from the chemo and I was hoping I would be one of these, although I knew it would be unlikely. About 10 days after my first chemo, I was sitting in my chair watching TV. My ex-husband was sitting on the couch. I brushed my fingers through my hair and a handful of hair came out. My heart sank. I looked at Darrel and said "I think I am losing my hair" as my eyes filled with tears. Losing my breast didn't really bother me. No one could see it and I was single so it was no big deal. Losing my hair, which was very visible, and a big part of who I was, was a big deal. The wigs were in my room waiting to be used and I had a feeling it would not be too long before they too became a part of me. Each morning I woke up, my pillow was full of hair and my scalp was becoming more visible.

At my second chemo session, the nurse commented on how my hair was thinning. I tried to play it down but it really bothered me that she noticed and commented on it. To her, it was probably nothing and just conversation, but to me it was my hair and I didn't want to lose it. A couple of days after my second chemo session, I looked in the mirror and decided that I was going to be the one to decide when I am bald and that time was now. I got the scissors out of the drawer, cut my hair as close to the scalp as I could and then finished the job with my razor. It felt good being in control. I was the one who decided the fate of my hair, not the chemo. This was a moment of triumph. There was no need for me to feel sorry for myself. I was alive and had a great family who loved me. What more could I ask for? Out came the wig and all of a sudden I had a full head of hair again.

The next couple of chemo sessions weren't too bad at all. Although I felt a little cuckoo for a couple of days afterwards, it didn't stop me from doing the things I wanted to do. I went shopping with my friend Gill to buy a shed and the two of us put it together the day of chemo. My sister and her family came over from England and we went to Disneyland, even taking my wig off to go on some of the rides. I recall coming off a ride and proceeding to the exit, where the pictures were displayed of people on the ride. A group of later teenage boys were there laughing at the faces and one of them commented "look at the bald chick". I looked at them, with my wig now back on and said "Isn't she beautiful". They gave me the strangest look and walked away. I had no reason to feel embarrassed and those boys had no idea why that lady in the picture was bald. Whether it was from choice or not, they had no idea and should not comment on people's appearances. From that point on, I walked around with my head held high and if I felt hot and sticky and my wig was irritating me, I took it off. There was nothing wrong with being bald. I was beautiful.

Each day I began to feel stronger and more confident that I was going to come out of this ordeal a winner. Ten weeks after my first chemo, I did a cancer walk and was proud to wear the "survivor" ribbon. My girls did the walk with me and were no longer afraid to come near me or touch me. Several of my friends who had also had breast cancer also walked and half of my daughter's 8th grade class joined us. What a day this was. A little over six months since I had the mammogram which identified my cancer and now my treatment was complete. I could get on with my life.

My hair gradually began to grow back. I was sitting in the computer room when my youngest daughter walked in and then immediately left. That was a little strange, but I didn't think too much of it. All of a sudden I felt a little pain on my head. "Ouch!" I said kind of loudly and looked around to see Jille standing there with tweezers in her hand. She had seen this one little lonely hair and was wondering if it would come out easy like my hair had been doing. This hair was solid though and did hurt when it came out. Although I was a little irritated at her pulling out my only hair, it was also a nice feeling knowing that my hair no longer came out easy and without feeling. I was returning to old me, minus one hair for now.

Here I sit, nine years later, and the cancer is just a memory. I still go for my regular check ups and yearly mammograms and September 2015 will be my 10-year mark. Cancer is a horrible disease and it is extremely important for women to be aware of their body and how it feels. If something feels different or not right, make an appointment to see your doctor and have it checked. My body felt odd and something was telling me that there was something wrong, even though I did not have any lumps or discharge. Being persistent and helping direct my medical care helped diagnose the cancer early and possibly saved my life. An uplifting book I read was "Chicken Soup for the Breast Cancer Survivor" which was a compilation of many different stories of women who had breast cancer. Women were made to be strong to raise their children and we can get through anything, even cancer.

After I had my biopsy, I decided I was going to keep a scrapbook of my journey, beginning with the pictures of how my breast looked at that moment in time. This was quite a therapeutic project and I added as much humor to it as I could. Although having cancer was scary, I always kept a positive outlook and tried not to let the fact that I had it dictate my life and how I was going to live at that time. It did impose some minor restrictions, but not many, and once I decided I was in control of the situation the restrictions went away.

A friend of mine gave me a piece of paper with a verse on it about cancer when I was first diagnosed and I keep this on my refrigerator all of the time.

Mary L. Maas

What Cancer Cannot Do

Cancer is so limited
It cannot cripple love
It cannot shatter hope
It cannot corrode faith
It cannot destroy peace
It cannot kill friendship
It cannot suppress memories
It cannot silence courage
It cannot invade the soul
It cannot steal eternal life
It cannot conquer the spirit!
I got cancer, it didn't get me.

Chapter Four

Alice Herbolsheimer

I was diagnosed in January of 1997, when my doctor found a lump during my regular yearly breast exam. I was given the choice of a lumpectomy, if the cancer was "in situ", or a mastectomy, if the cancer had spread. He said if the cancer had not spread to the lymph nodes, he was hopeful that with a mastectomy, I would not need further treatment.

My husband and family were there for me, amidst many tears, as the "C" word is huge and scary. I had no relatives with breast cancer, to my knowledge. I read everything I could find that might help us through this. For my follow-up treatment, I took an oral chemotherapy pill for five years, with very few side effects.

Looking back at my experience, I probably would not do anything differently today. It has been over fifteen years since I was diagnosed. The doctor told me to be careful of the deodorants I used, as it is good for my body to get rid of the toxins by sweating some. He also said the first chance I got after work, or whenever, to remove my bra or wear a sports bra, because he said it also helps to get rid of toxins without a binding bra.

My best encouragement for others would be sure to get your annual checkup and don't neglect to do your monthly self-exam of your breasts. I take one day at a time. I feel now I am much more sensitive to others with similar problems. I have been very thankful that all has gone well for me so far, and I keep praying for good health to continue.

Chapter Five

Elaine Roessle

It was May 5, 2011. Cinco de Mayo. She wouldn't look me in the eye – and I knew. The flailing shred of hope we clung to was lost in that moment. "Come with me," she said, and we did. "The doctor will be with you shortly," she told us. Again with no eye contact. Bracing ourselves for what was to come, my husband and I sat holding hands awaiting the confirmation. Seconds felt like hours as we waited, our minds racing yet still trying to cling to an innocent shred of hope that we misread her body language.

Enter the doctor. He, too, avoided eye contact as he confirmed the biopsy results – Breast Cancer. Inflammatory Breast Cancer, triple negative – the worst and most aggressive kind. This couldn't be happening. There is no history of any kind of cancer in my family.

"Am I terminal?" I asked him. He kept his head down, shrugged his shoulders and told us to follow him as he led us down to Oncology. He got us in to see the oncologist immediately, no more waiting. That can't be good. It's that urgent? Don't they usually set up appointments and try to get you in "ASAP". They don't escort you down there.

I barely remember that first visit with the oncologist. I do, however, remember that she was very kind and very concerned. We didn't have insurance. I've had insurance my entire life up to that point. The recession hit us hard and we had to lay off the three employees we had to run the business which left just us, my husband and me. That also meant giving up the business insurance plan. We tried to secure private insurance, but having asthma put me in a high risk category, and they wanted $1,800 a month for coverage. We simply didn't have that. The medical oncologist insisted we had to start chemotherapy immediately. There was no time to wait to find insurance of some sort. She could contact Count (OMG!), or we could start there.

We started and they worked out a payment plan for us – we'll be paying that off for the rest of our lives, no doubt. We didn't ask for a prognosis at that point. I didn't want to know anymore. Something clicked in my head, a survival mode of some sort, and I decided then and there that dying from this wasn't an option. Having stat's or time frames and percentages would do me no good. They'd only place doubt and fear in my mind.

My husband lost his mother to cancer as a young teen. It brought him to his knees. Losing his wife to cancer also just wasn't going to happen as far as I was concerned. I would fight for him, too.

My treatment plan: Six months of neoadjuvant chemotherapy, a mastectomy, and then six weeks of radiation. It was grueling, but with the love and support of my family and friends, I muscled through it. My husband shaved my head while my son held my hand, offering to shave his own head in solidarity. I didn't let him. I did everything I could to stay positive during chemo. I read books on getting well, the power of positive thinking. I watched The Ellen Show religiously and laughed at every single thing I could, our rescue dogs by my side.

The six months felt like six years, but they finally came to an end. My husband and friends surprised me with a day at the spa to celebrate the end of the chemo. It was exactly what I needed. My husband gave me the most beautiful birthday card. I have it framed in a shadow box. It says, "I'm so glad I found you. If I had my life to live over again, next time I'd find you sooner, so I could love you longer." Then he wrote how much he loves me and how he's looking forward to many, many years. Be still my heart. He's a keeper for sure. How did I get so lucky?

After a break to recover from the chemo, I underwent a radical mastectomy right before Thanksgiving. My family and friends, once again, rallied around us. Soon after, I was feeling well enough to attend one of my son's basketball games. I decided to wear a mastectomy camisole I had bought that had a pocket for the fake breast. My husband and I stood in line to buy our tickets and the young man taking our money was staring at me, blatantly, like something was wrong. I thought perhaps my wig was askew and he was noticing. I tried to straighten the wig and we went to our seats.

After the game, we returned home and once I was in the bathroom, I finally knew what the young man was staring at – my camisole had shifted and my fake breast was almost under my chin. I had tears in my eyes from laughing so hard. You know you've been married a long time when your husband doesn't even notice that!!

In January, 2013, I started daily radiation for six weeks. It was a cakewalk compared to the chemotherapy. My skin reacted badly. I had open oozing wounds, but that is a small price to pay for a life-saving treatment. The nurse did daily dressing and it soon healed. It was now March, 2013, and I was declared in remission.

WOW. I did it. I kicked cancer's butt. Eight months later, I am still reeling from that realization. It makes me feel stronger and more powerful,

I learned that it it's not the things in life, it's the people, pets and experiences and am grateful to cancer for reminding me of that.

My original decision to have reconstructive surgery has changed. The radiation treatments made having the flap surgery a necessity. I would have donor skin from my back to be added to the breast; an expander inserted and five to six months of saline injections. This would be followed by another surgery to remove the expander and put in the permanent implant. Then I had another surgery, with more donor skin for the areola and nipple. I have decided at this point, that I don't want to go ahead with it. There's too much living to do and I don't want to miss a moment of it.

Chapter Six

Barbara J. (Boyd) Wolverton

I was 41 when I was diagnosed with breast cancer, on May 12, 2005. I have three daughters and a husband. I found the lump in my right breast in January of that year; I didn't get it checked out until April. My husband's father was dying from stage four lung and esophagus cancer, and things were pretty rough for us. My father–in-law had been given only six months to live and things were moving fast. I figured my lump was probably an enlarged milk duct or cyst. My sister had some of those, so I didn't think too much about it. I chose to ignore it for the time being. Not a good choice.

In March, my husband's paternal grandmother became ill and died very suddenly. My family was grieving her death as we were watching my husband's father's health deteriorate more and more.

I still had the lump in my breast and decided that I needed to get it checked out. I scheduled an appointment to see my gynecologist for a mammogram. A few days before my appointment, my father-in-law died. It had only been a few weeks since his own mother's death. My family was not in a very good emotional state at this point. My young daughters were completely heartbroken to lose two grandparents so close together. My husband and I were devastated to lose two strong pillars of our family.

I knew I needed to go ahead to my doctor appointment and I had an ultrasound and mammogram of my breast. After viewing the x-rays, the radiologist suggested that I needed to have a stereotactic biopsy of the lump. A couple days later I had the test done and waited for the results. Two weeks after my father-in-law's death, I was called by the radiologist and told that I had breast cancer. He told me that I needed to find a surgeon. I was scared to death. One thing that sticks in my mind is what my youngest daughter, who was only five, said when we told her that I had cancer. She said, "Well, great grandma had cancer and died and grandpa had cancer and died and now you'll die, and who will take care of us?" Instead of telling her that I wasn't going to die, I told her that she had lots of people that loved her and would take care of her. I wish now that I would have realized that I needed to tell her that I wasn't going to die, but at that time, I was scared that I wasn't thinking that way. I, too, thought I was going to die.

The time after that day seemed to speed crazily by. I met with a surgeon and got a second opinion from another surgeon. Both agreed that I needed to have surgery. One choice that I was able to make was if I wanted to do chemotherapy before the surgery to try and shrink the tumor, or to have chemotherapy after surgery. I chose to try Neo-adjuvant chemo (chemo that is given before surgery). I was hoping that it would shrink the tumor enough that I would only have to have a lumpectomy, rather than a mastectomy.

When I had my port put in to get my chemo through, I also had a sentinel node removal. It showed that the cancer had metastasized to that first lymph node under my arm. I found a wonderful group of oncologists who worked together on finding the best route for me to take. I was assured that doing the chemo before the surgery was not going to make a difference for the cancer spreading further during that time. The nurses at this clinic were also wonderful and I became good friends with them. I can't lie and say that chemo was easy, it wasn't. It was the hardest thing I have ever done and it made me feel like I was 100 years old. The doctors said since I was diagnosed at a young age, they were going to "sock it to" the cancer and give me some very powerful stuff. They did.

I was so tired on many days that just getting up and going down the stairs in my house was a challenge. My days and night just seemed to blend together. I took chemo from June until September. I had some time to recoup from the chemo and get my white blood count back up before having surgery. The tumor did not shrink as much as I and the doctors were hoping it might, so I ended up having a complete mastectomy. My surgeon said his gut instinct was telling him that was what he needed to do. I trusted his opinion and knowledge and it turned out that I was correct in doing so. When the testing of the mastectomy tissue came back, the cancer was sprinkled throughout many places of the breast tissue. The margins were clear though and I didn't have to have any other surgery to remove more tissue. I was relieved about that. Now I could get on with the healing of my body and spirit. The physical recovery of the surgery was not a nearly as bad as going through the chemotherapy. Everything was starting to look better.

On October 18, 2005, I was told by my surgeon that my cancer was gone. He was confident that they had gotten it all. Never in my life have I been so relieved and thankful than I was on that day. It is so ironic that day was also the birth date of my father-in-law. Yes, I do believe in angels!

So here I am eight years later, still alive and kicking! I don't get as nervous as I used to when I go to my annual oncology appointment. I get a better sense of security with every year that passes. I even made up my mind to go through with reconstructive surgery. I had a DIEP flap done and I'm very pleased with the results. I still have a couple smaller surgeries to do, but the hardest part is done. It was very tough for the first several weeks as I was told by the doctor it would be. There were a few times that I had wondered if I had made the right choice, but when I take a quick peek down my shirt and see that I have a breast again on my right side, after not having one for eight years, I get this overwhelming feeling of being whole again. It was a good decision for me, even if it took me a while to get the courage and confidence to commit to it.

I have a great support system consisting of family and friends, who have made this journey much easier for me. When I was first diagnosed eight years ago, a friend and cancer survivor told me to let people help you when they offer and to not be too proud or stubborn to accept. Then he said, "When you're better, 'you pass it on' to the next person when they need it." It was some of the best advice I was given.

This is why I agreed to tell my story. I'm hoping that at least one person realizes that this is beatable and that no matter how scared and worried you are at the time, things will work out. Keep your faith in yourself and surround yourself with positive people. I never once let anyone tell me any negative stories that happened to them or someone they knew. Yes, there were a couple times where I felt that was the way a conversation was going, so I would simply say that I didn't want to hear anything negative and that would do the trick of changing the subject. It is way too easy to get down and it is way too hard to build that confidence back up once you are down, so don't let anyone take your positive thoughts away from you. You can do it!

Chapter Seven

Jo Mandl

My life and that of my family changed forever on June 23, 2011. A routine diabetic doctor's appointment turned into a complete physical. Eventually, the doctor asked who my surgeon was. Why? He had found a lump. Cancer, not me! I hadn't felt a lump and I just had a mammogram in September of 2010. That mammogram was normal. I figured it was just another fibrocystic lump. No problem, I thought, the results usually come back benign.

Now, how I would break the news about the possibility of cancer to my husband. Of course, it came as a total shock. You never imagine it happening to you. We knew that we had to go in to it with a positive attitude and we were going to take one day at a time if it turned out to be cancer. We decided not to tell our daughter until we knew for sure.

The surgeon wanted an ultrasound done of the left breast first. What a shock when the radiologist said that it was cancer! A biopsy was ordered to confirm his findings. Now, we had to tell our daughter, granddaughters and the rest of our family the news. Total shock for them, too. But, I knew in my heart that my very special guardian angel, our son Scott, and God would watch over me. One day at a time and lots of prayers from family and friends would help me through this.

More tests were ordered. After the biopsy confirmed the malignancy, a lumpectomy was ordered immediately. This would remove the tumor and a sentinel lymph node. Results from that confirmed that the cancer had spread to the lymph nodes and more cancer cells were found in the tissue that had been sent in.

My next option, in August, was a modified radical mastectomy and more lymph nodes needed to be removed on the left side. I wanted the right breast removed at the same time, but "Obama Care" and insurance stated that this was an unnecessary procedure. After the mastectomy, the lab results showed more cancer cells in some of the lymph nodes and more in the tissue.

I was diagnosed with Stage 3a Lobular Carcinoma. The size of the tumor was about 3 inches. My medical oncologist told us that he was going to hit this hard and try to save my life.

Chemotherapy and radiation would follow as soon as I was healed from the mastectomy surgery. My veins are what they call "floating veins" which means they move when inserting a needle, so I choose to have a port implanted. The port made it easier to receive the drugs and all the blood work that would follow.

I was given chemotherapy that they refer to as Kool-Aid, because of its color, RED! The drugs are known as AC (doxorubicin and cyclophosphamide). This form of chemo prevents cancer cells from splitting and growing and can help the cancer cells to shrink and die. It could damage the heart muscle and cause heart failure, so I had to have a MUGA (Multiple Gated Acquisition Scan) scan done. Before the scan, a technician drew blood from my arm and he added a trace amount of radioactive tracer to the blood he had withdrawn. This was injected into a vein. I was then told to lie on a table and the gamma camera went to work. This camera focused on the radioactive red blood cells going through the chambers of my heart. I passed! My heart was healthy enough to receive the AC chemotherapy.

Usually, this form of chemotherapy is given at three weeks intervals, but because of the aggression of my cancer, I was given it every other week. Blood tests monitored my health before each treatment. Along with the chemo, I was given anti-nausea meds before the treatment. My treatment sessions took around three hours to complete. Twenty-four hours later, I was given a shot to help keep my white-blood cell count up. Also, the medical oncologist ordered two anti-nausea prescriptions to be taken at home. One, I used twice a day for five days after the chemotherapy treatment and the other was to be used as needed.

My first chemotherapy treatment was the worst. The lab tests showed that I was low on blood (possibly from all the surgeries), so I had to have two units of blood the next day, along with my shot. I didn't feel well for about three or four days after this. By the time it was ready for the next treatment, I was feeling much better.

Yes, the hair started to fall out after the first treatment, so I had my husband shave my hair off. We joked that he now had more hair than me. I used hats and scarves to protect my head. Wigs didn't look right or feel right for me. Our daughter and granddaughters always seemed to supply me with hats.

The following AC treatments left me tired, but not nauseous. I was able to keep up with some things around the house. I tried to keep up with the washing and dishes. If the dusting or vacuuming didn't get done, so what! My husband made meals when I wasn't up to it. My daughter and her girls would make meals and bring them out to us. Of course, we would go out for breakfast on the days of chemo.

Here I was 60 years old and going through all this. Whenever I felt sorry for myself, my thoughts would always go back to a child dealing with cancer; I really didn't have it so bad. I lived a full life, but they had so much more to experience in life. My younger sister had gone through cancer treatments seventeen years earlier and her experience was totally different. Treatment of cancer has changed so dramatically over the years.

Following the two months of AC treatments, I needed to have twelve weekly treatments of another chemo drug (Paclitaxel/Taxol). This meant more weekly blood tests and an additional drug (Dexamethasone) was given to prevent an allergic reaction to the chemo drug prior to the treatments. Benadryl was added to counteract the restless leg syndrome I developed during these treatments. These twelve weeks left me totally drained.

In December 2011, I developed a blood clot in my right lung. Blood clots are one of the side effects of the chemo treatments. I had to have several shots of Arixtra to thin my blood. After that, I was given warfarin to regulate my pro-time.

Following the completion of my chemotherapy the middle of January, I suffered several side effects. Tests were done to see if there was any damage to my system from the chemo. I lost 20% of my bone density, my mitral valve in my heart is now prolapsed and I have chemo-induced neuropathy. I take more calcium and have to have a Prolia shot twice a year for the bone density. My cardiologist keeps an eye on my mitral valve. I am on Lyrica for the neuropathy. The medical oncologist said that the chemo would stay in my system for a year.

February 2012, I was now ready for my radiation treatments. We met with the radiation oncologist; he explained the side effects of radiation and informed us that I needed to have thirty-five sessions. The radiation would be given at the site of the cancer. These treatments were a breeze compared to the chemo sessions. It took longer to undress for radiation than it did for the actual treatment. I felt lucky, because I suffered very little skin reaction to the radiation. My neck was a little sore, but that was from the collar of the clothing rubbing on the area hit by radiation. Wherever the radiation was aimed, my skin is now darker. I completed my radiation treatments the end of March, 2012.

I go back to the oncologist every three months for lab work. This tells me if my cancer is in remission or not. The last marker test was done in September showed very little sign of cancer in my body. I return the end of this month for another marker test. The time period between the marker tests will vary at the discretion of my medical oncologist. Eventually, the tests will be done once yearly.

I am looking forward to my reconstructive surgery now. I chose not to have it right after the mastectomy. All the research I read convinced me that radiation may cause damage to the implant or that it may not properly reach the area that the radiation was intended for. This is a decision that one must make for herself/himself. Yes, men can get breast cancer also.

As for my hair, it is slowly coming back in. Amazing, it is coming back in the same color (salt and pepper) as it was before the chemo. My strength is slowly coming back. I still have my bad days, especially when I overdo it. But with the help of my family, all the prayers and my belief in God and my guardian angel, I am looking at being cancer-free for years to come.

Chapter Eight

Terry Warnke

I always do a monthly breast examination as a habit. With my experience as a licensed practical nurse, I know the importance of doing this procedure, to palpate the breast and check for lumps. In July of 1995, I was showering to get ready for work. I found a lump as I was doing my self-examination. "What is this", I said to myself. I rechecked the lump again and again. "It must be a hormonal thing", I thought. I had been told there's no breast cancer in my family history. So I put the knowledge of the lump aside as I went off to work. However, I kept it in mind to watch this lump and watch for any changes.

In July of 1995, I had some plans, some great plans. I was asked by my girlfriend, Margaret, to go to Korea with her and her son John to gather up her grandchildren. They were in Korea with their mother, who was stationed there in the United States Air Force. Margaret's daughter, Donna, wanted her children stateside to start school when the school session started. Donna wouldn't finish her tour in Korea until October. I wanted to go to Korea with my friend for my own reasons.

My daughter-in-law, Eunah, is Korean and I wanted to go see her culture and meet her mother. Eunah was happy for me to make this trip and encouraged me to go. Eunah wasn't able to go along with me, so she made arrangements for me to meet her mother and tried to find me an interpreter. My son, Todd, was stationed in Yongsun, Korea in the United States Army for two years and that's how he met Eunah. Todd wanted to know about Korea culture and Eunah wanted to improve her English. I wanted to go to Korea. I felt this was a good opportunity to go and see my daughter- in-law's country, and meet her mother. I would see what Todd saw when he was in Korea

In the meantime, this new lump I found wasn't my top priority. My journey to Korea was heavenly and I was glad I went. When I returned home from the trip to Korea, I returned to my routine of going to work and doing things for my family. I kept monitoring this lump. I don't remember mentioning this lump to my family.

I always do my yearly mammogram in October. Not only is this the month for Breast cancer awareness, it is also my birthday. I felt these dates were good to remember to get my mammogram done. I made an appointment to have my mammogram done the first of October. On the day of the examination, I went in early in the morning. I noticed the technician was taking several pictures and had me reposition my body better so she could get a better view. When she finished, she told me to go ahead and get dressed, but she asked me to wait. She wanted the radiologist to look at the mammogram x-rays. When she came back to the room she asked if I could go for an ultrasound. In my heart I knew this was not going to be good. I told the technician that I needed to call my family to tell them I was going to be late.

I called my husband, Clint, and told him what was going on. I mainly needed to have his support and a strong arm to hold me with even the thought that the lump might be cancerous. My mind was rushing. How is Clint going to handle this news? Just a year ago he lost his younger sister, Wynnette to this disease. But my husband was a rock and he came to the hospital just to be there for me.

When the sonogram was finished, the technician told me I should go to my primary doctor. I told them that my nurse practitioner ordered this test, but the tech told me I must see a medical doctor. They arranged an appointment to see a doctor. The physician reviewed the test and ordered a needle biopsy. The biopsy was scheduled the next day.

The rest of the day I was in a whirl, lots of 'what ifs', 'what I am going to do', and 'is this the right thing to do'. Finally my mind let go of all these thoughts and I was going take what the next day was going to bring.

The next morning started out with my whole demeanor being on edge. From my sleepless night and several prayers, my nerves were running amok. I wanted to get this procedure done and see what is going on in my body. During a needle biopsy, they take a hollow needle and insert into the lump and aspirate fluid or tissue from the lump in the breast. At the hospital I had to remove my upper clothing and I was instructed to lay face down on the table. The table had an opening to place my exposed breast through. My vision was obstructed, my head facing the table. I couldn't see what was going on, in a matter of time I felt a snap, snap as the needle was removing the needed tissue. The procedure didn't cause any pain. I was uncomfortable being tied down to this table, I felt powerless, lying on the table, feeling the snip, snip as the procedure went on and on. While lying on the table with my breast inside of the hole, my thoughts went back to the farm. When I was a little girl, I remembered how the cows were drawn into the stall. Their heads were penned in so they couldn't escape while they waited to be milked. After what seemed like forever, the procedure was finished. All the tech said was I could get dressed.

The tissue would be sent to the pathologist and I should hear from my physician the next day. I went home, not feeling elated with all the things I had to go through with the needle biopsy. I was glad it was over.

That night my husband Clint, daughter Tyra, and granddaughter, Tessa, spent a very solemn evening and night. The next day I heard from my doctor, the result was what we all expected "cancerous tumor grade 3"

"I WANT TO GET RID OF THIS!"

My surgery was scheduled for Oct 9, the same day as my 50th birthday. It was amazing how calm I was, at least that what I thought, I don't know how the family was feeling. When I become aware of my surroundings, after being under anesthesia, I reached under my cover and noted the bandages and a very flat surface. It is gone! The nasty cancer is gone!

When my family came to see me at the hospital, I felt so fortunate to have a loving and caring husband, sons and daughter who were so supportive, which helped me heal. Many of my friends were there to support me, too.

After leaving the hospital and going home, Tyra was my main caregiver. She took over the responsibility to make the meals, do the shopping, and other errands. When my wounds healed and no longer needed the drainage tubes, the doctor told me I needed six months of chemotherapy as extra precaution. I was told after the surgery that they got everything, but they felt chemotherapy will definitely detain the possible growth of any cancerous cells.

Six long months of chemotherapy made me very sick. I went to have the chemotherapy every two weeks. One Wednesday, I went home with a queasy stomach. I felt fatigued and was losing my hair. (I thought I could actually hear my hair follicles falling out each day.) The second week after chemotherapy was done, I got stronger every day. Then it was time to go back for more chemotherapy.

I didn't lose all my hair, just had straggles of hair, some here and there--I looked like a plucked chicken (there I go back to my farm days). Within a year my hair grew back in full. HAPPY ME!!! I felt in time I could get a permanent, which I did. It was so spirit-lifting to look better. There's something to be said about having a good hair day.

In June of 1996 I became a grandmother again. No more thoughts of sickness. My hair was coming back and I had my new grandson to enjoy. Eben, what a boy, and what a joy. No more chemotherapy. Life was good.

I wore prosthesis for a time and hated it. The prosthesis tended to wander or float around my chest. I looked lop-sided and was uncomfortable to be out in public. I was forever putting the prosthesis in place.

Two years later they found a cancerous mass in my other breast. Because of my past cancer history, the doctor talked me into having surgery. Since the cancer hadn't spread into my lymph nodes, I didn't have to have the chemotherapy. YEAH!!!

As time passed, I decided to go back for breast implants. That is the best surgery for those who have a mastectomy. I'm glad I had it done.

Now I am in my eighteenth year as a cancer survivor. That is good news for me. Not for my sister Judi. She found a lump in her breast and kept it secret from her family. The lump in her breast grew and later it broke. She doctored it herself, kept it bandaged and went on with her life. Later when she had some stomach problems, she went to a doctor. While there, she told the doctor about her other problems and showed him the drainage from her breast. He told her that it was probably cancer. My sister didn't want to go through all the tests to confirm the diagnosis. She didn't have health insurance, and she didn't have the money for surgery and treatment, so she let it go. When she finally told me about her cancer, we made arrangements for comfort care. In one month after I found out about her cancer, she was gone... I miss her so much. In hindsight I wish I had known what was going on in her life and maybe things could have turned out as well as it has for me.

I really am thankful to my heavenly Father and my family and friends. I couldn't have gone through this illness without them.

Chapter Nine

Charlie

My story begins in the month of June of 2010. Yes the famous month for my dreaded yearly checkup. I had felt a lump once again. I found a lump in my left breast back in 1969, when I was 19 years old. The doctor felt the round cyst about the size of a golf ball during my exam. He said to me, "That shouldn't be in there." Being naïve and only in my teens, I never even thought of cancer. So, I was not afraid that it was anything serious. I had surgery on a Friday and the cyst turned out to be a B9 – negative.

I went back to work on Monday and I was glad it was all over, but I was left with a big scar on my breast. Life went on and I got married in 1971. I have three boys and nursed two of them without any problems.

In March of 1979, my dad died of lung cancer and in 1995, my father-in-law died from throat cancer. That's when I took the thought of cancer more seriously. So, I had my annual mammograms done without complaints.

Then in 2000, my mammogram came back abnormal. I had calcifications that had formed and there was a cluster of three in one area towards the front of my left breast. I had thirteen calcifications removed in the office that day. The doctor told me he'd put in a small metal piece, where the cluster had formed, to keep an eye on that spot in the future. None of the calcifications tested positive for cancer. That was one procedure I did not want to have done again. It was painful and it took me a few weeks to not be sore and to be able to use my left arm normally again.

Our first grandson was born that month and we bought tickets to Virginia to see him. I cried and thanked God that it wasn't cancer once again. All was good for many years.

In March, 2009, my son and I were in a hit-and-run accident. The seatbelt really tightened on my left breast and left me bruised. I should have had it checked immediately, but I didn't. I didn't go in for my mammogram in June that year as our fourth grandchild was born that month. Our daughter-in-law's father was diagnosed with cancer behind his ear and had to take chemotherapy and radiation treatments, so my mammogram was forgotten.

I wish now I hadn't been too busy to go and have one done. In May of 2010, I noticed a lump and made an appointment for a physical in June. I thought it was another cyst, though it felt a little different than the first one did in 1969. It was located where the three calcifications were marked in 2000. Still, I was not too worried, but I should have been as my primary doctor didn't feel it during the exam. So, I pointed it out to her and she said she didn't know what it was, but she would set up a diagnostic mammogram. H-m-m-m-m! That should have set off a warning for me. I went to have the mammogram test and when they found something wrong, I was sent in for an ultrasound, again on my left breast.

The doctor wanted a sample of the lump. After I was dressed, my doctor came in to see me. I knew he had bad news. He was very nice even when he told me cancer can be cured. He would not look me directly in the eye.

For some reason, I knew in my heart I would be okay. So I smiled and told him, too, I would be okay. He had this look like "she is not hearing me". But, I had heard him and I went out and told my husband they found something.

We waited for my primary doctor to call and fortunately, I received it on my husband's day off. We both went in to get the news that it was indeed cancer. The lump measured two centimeters and we were told the whole breast needed to be removed with follow-up chemotherapy.

I remembered what my dad and father-in-law went through with chemo treatments and I was not ready for that. I had another grandchild on the way and due in December. I was scheduled with a breast cancer specialist and surgeon for appointments right away that month. I met with her and she examined the lump. She said the lump was quite large; however it was only in Stage One and not an aggressive form of cancer. I received a diagnosis of Invasive Ductal Carcinoma. I had the choice of a full or partial mastectomy. The doctor, my husband and I decided the choice would be a partial mastectomy. The doctor said there wasn't much difference in the two surgeries when it came to removal of the cancer and I would have to have reconstruction done by a plastic surgeon afterwards. We chose a doctor who could perform plastic and reconstructive surgery at either hospital in Sioux Falls. He said he preferred not to do a breast reduction on my right breast at the same. Then I was given a packet on breast cancer and I could keep my insurance papers, appointment cards, and a year's diary for appointments and comments all in the same packet.

The date for surgery was scheduled and we went to see the surgeon in July. I had before pictures and measurements taken, which was rather embarrassing.

My surgery was scheduled for August 6th, 2010. All the waiting, worrying and appointments were getting to me by this time. It was taking forever to get the lump removed and I was worried about the lump growing bigger all the while I waited.

If it hadn't been for my husband, who was my rock and the one who shared my tears, plus all my family and friends supporting me, I couldn't have faced the surgery and climbed the mountains that rose before me.

On the day of surgery, I had to be at the hospital at 5 a.m. to be ready for surgery at 7 a.m. I was taken to pre-op to put on a gown and socks, and then they started an I.V. They gave me two pain pills and described what I would have done in surgery. The surgeon came in and said her part of the surgery would take about four hours. Then the plastic surgeon came in to mark my breast, while I was standing, to do the reconstruction part and make sure it was done on the correct breast! Then he drew a sad face on my left breast. He was trying to reassure me and said his part of the surgery would be finished in about two hours. Now we were talking about six hours of surgery. A nurse came in with a numbing cream and said I would have six to eight shots so they could shoot dye into my lymph nodes to be able to check them for any cancer cells. Then I went to an x-ray room where I had to lay on a very narrow, metal table. I was sure I would fall off and I said to the two nurses, "You're kidding, right?" They both smiled and helped me on and off the table after I was given the shots. Thank heaven for the numbing crème and the pain pills because the shots were still a bit painful. Then they wheeled me out to my hubby to tell him that I would see him in six hours.

I was to hurry through the double doors where more nurses waited to put me up on another dang narrow, metal table! They said they had to hurry as the dye only lasted about twenty minutes. The table made my back hurt, so they put a pillow beneath my knees. That was the last I knew and I was out.

My surgery went so well, that in two hours it was over, and then I spent another hour in recovery. I had to stay in the hospital overnight for observation and pain control. I had good nurses and saw both doctors in the afternoon. They were pleased with the way the surgery went and that the cancer had not spread to the lymph nodes. They sent the tissue to California to a lab for analysis to determine whether I needed both chemotherapy and radiation treatments and for how long. I would have to wait a month to heal. Then I had doctor appointments scheduled for a two week checkup. At that time, I would meet another doctor for my radiation schedule, every day, five days a week, for six weeks. I would see the radiation doctor once a week during the treatments for him to follow my progress in handling radiation and for checking my skin for any signs of irritation.

I was blessed with eight tattooed dots for my first visit with the radiologist and had to have a bone density test. The radiation treatment lasted about five minutes and I did tolerate them quite well, though my stomach was upset after about the first 10 treatments. This also made me quite fatigued and I would take an hour long nap after the radiation. Everything was well until the booster treatment phase for the final five visits. The booster phase concentrates the radiation directly to the location where the cancer grew. On the third day I became quite ill and slept for several hours. When I awoke, very early the following morning, I had pain in my left breast and it felt like there were bubbles circling around the area of the scar. I wasn't able to see the doctor until 11:00 a.m. By that time I was in so much pain, I thought maybe I was having a heart attack, so my husband took me to Emergency. After a short wait, I had tests, an X-Ray and an IV started for preliminary care, but the pain increased and I was given pain medication with the IV. They didn't work fast enough, and though I have a very high pain tolerance, by that time I was in tears. The pain was more than I could handle. Even after the meds kicked in, I remained at a five to six grade level of pain and I could still feel the bubbling sensation. The doctor came in with my chart in his hand and he greeted me with the statement, "Well, if you had to have cancer, you got the good kind!" I didn't know there was a good kind! Then he told me I had a reaction to the radiation and it wouldn't be the last time, and he promptly walked out of my room. Needless to say, I was not very pleased with him. The nurses called the radiation clinic across the street to alert them as to where I was, and that I would be late for my radiation treatment! They still wanted me to have a radiation treatment when I was so wiped out from the reaction! I had only two treatments left, so I finished out, and fortunately, I did not have any more problems.

In November, I had appointments with two doctors for checkups and then I met a new doctor who would do the follow-ups with blood tests and an examination every six months for the next five years.

At the end of January in 2011, I had a breast reduction performed on my right breast to make it match the left side. That was outpatient surgery which went quite well and I went home that afternoon. Unfortunately, that wound didn't heal well and I developed an infection in a couple of the stitches. I found out that infection can happen due to your immune system being lowered after radiation, so I had to take antibiotics for two months. If I had it to do over, I would have had the breast reduction performed during my lumpectomy.

I was also told to take Vitamin D-3, a multi-vitamin and fish oil twice a day, plus ibuprofen or Tylenol, when needed. I was given a prescription for a daily dose of Anastrozole (Arimidex) for five years.

I am two years out now and free of cancer. I still am fatigued, my joints ache more and my sex drive is next to nil. These are all side effects that can be from that one small Arimidex pill. I still get a pulling pain by the scar on my left breast which can take my breath away for a few seconds. The scars are no longer a bright pink, but are more natural skin color. The doctors think everything is doing well. I do notice on cold days and on stormy days, my left breast will ache more than usual and I wear something loose to relieve that pain.

My sister was diagnosed with breast cancer a year after I finished my radiation treatments. I tried to help her through the first part as cancer is a very scary word for anyone. The treatments and cures have come a long way and bring much more hope for positive outcomes. Still, today, all the advertisements can get to me because they remind me that I had cancer, and that is something I prefer to forget. I would like to forget it all for a while, but I never do really. Every day I thank God for being with me. My life changed a lot and I feel it changed to be better. I see things differently than I did before. I don't take things for granted like I used to. I pray every night that cancer won't come back.

Some of us weren't fortunate to have escaped cancer, but with the workshops, meetings, family and friends for support, we can make it through.

This is my story. I still have three years to go with my six month checkups, mammograms, doctor appointments and blood tests. I can handle it, but I still get nervous on the days of my checkup. I am still afraid something will be spotted and something will not look normal. But, I always pray that won't happen.

Chapter Ten

Agnes Jeanette Hoagland

I was born in Yakima, Washington, 1938—and blessed with the name of Agnes Jeanette McDaniel. I married at age twenty and we raised six sons. All are now married with children of their own. My first attack from cancer arrived in 1993 with the screening of a routine mammogram. The doctor noted an abnormality in my right breast. My age at that time was fifty-five, with no family history of cancer. The doctor performed a needle localization biopsy—the results of which indicated a carcinoma. The surgical margins were free of tumor so a lumpectomy was recommended and accomplished. Armpit lymph nodes were also removed. My biopsy information was sent to The Virginia Mason Tumor Board in Seattle, Washington for their advice regarding continuing treatment. The Board recommended radiation therapy for a period of six weeks and to discontinue all replacement hormone supplements. Taking their suggestion I began treatments on approximately February 1, 1994.

At the time we lived in Port Angeles, Washington, which is located on the Olympic Peninsula, over a hundred miles west of Seattle by ferry and roadway. My husband accompanied me to each consultation and surgical treatment. We were required to go to Virginia Mason Hospital in Seattle in order to have a fitted form constructed to conform to the contours of my body. I received my radiation treatments in Port Angeles. For radiation, I would be positioned on my back—upon the form. Its only purpose to maintain my arms and shoulders in a correct position, allowing proper angles of the emission to be directed. It being quite uncomfortable, I was relieved to discover the treatments lasted less than a minute in length-of-time and my husband did not have to take time off from work to accompany me for the daily treatments each week.

To receive the last radiation treatment we drove to Seattle. This would be my final use of the positioning form and since it was uncomfortable to lie on, I was glad to be rid of it. The purpose of doing it in Seattle was because they could provide a more intensive radiation dosage. My husband and I were both greatly relieved when they gave that final treatment and I was finished with cancer treatments with the exception of healing. In time I was left with no pain, a puckered scar on my right breast and pronounced cancer free.

We had lived thirty years in Port Angeles when we sold our business and retired to Green Valley, Arizona in 2001. We lived in our large motor-home during the year our retirement home was being built. Delighted with the warm sunshine we took possession of our new home on September 10, 2001—one day before the destruction of the World Trade Center Twin Towers in New York City.

Life passed quickly as we made new friends and enjoyed the climate of southeast Arizona. Breast cancer became a forgotten memory. We went on cruises and traveled to far places in the world. Annual trips to Washington were taken to see our boys, their wives and the grandchildren.

It was December 2011 when I had a regular mammogram screening, which showed no abnormalities. Three weeks later on January 7, 2012, with self-examination, I discovered two lumps in the left breast. I saw my doctor on Wednesday, January 11th. She recommended an ultra-sound examination, which was done on Friday 13th. On Monday the 16th, lumps were confirmed and an appointment was set up for an MRI & biopsy on January 30, 2012.

On February 6, 2012—eighteen years and three months after being declared cancer-free—my primary doctor confirmed the presence of cancer in both lumps and set up an appointment with a surgeon at the University of Arizona Cancer Center, in Tucson, Arizona.

At a conference with the surgeon, a plan for treatment was laid out including surgery, blood tests and EKG—beginning February 13, 2012

On February 23rd I had a second MRI and ultrasound to determine exact location of tumors for surgery. On March 6th I had a third MRI, because of a shadow in the right breast discovered on the second MRI, which turned out to be of no concern. On March 9th surgery was performed on the left breast. At the post-op exam on March 19th, the surgeon explained that the margins on one lump were compromised, making it necessary to go back in and remove more surrounding tissue. The second surgery was accomplished on April 3rd. On April 9th, I met with the Oncology doctor to discuss chemotherapy treatments. It was decided there would be chemo treatments, once each week, lasting twenty weeks. Chemo treatments would be followed by six weeks of daily radiation therapy. My husband and I attended a chemotherapy education class at the Cancer Center—all subjects regarding the treatment of persons having breast cancer were discussed. We were amazed at the range of subjects covered, diet, psychological and physical effects—plus the exact procedures that would be taken during my treatment.

I chose to have a port inserted in my right chest near the shoulder. Since blood would have to be drawn in order to mix the chemo drugs injected on a weekly basis for twenty weeks, it would be much easier to draw from and inject into a port connected to a vein—instead of finding a new vein each week to draw blood from and another one to inject the medications into.

On April 30, 2012 the port was installed and I went for my first chemo treatment. They drew blood from the port, sent it to the lab where they produced the proper mix of drugs. The condition of the blood—its consistency, cells, etc—provides the information for the proper medication to be injected. Once the lab drew the blood it took approximately a half hour before the medication was ready. This was injected into the port, taking eight to ten minutes. My husband accompanied me for each visit, and from the time of arrival to departure from the Cancer Center usually lasted two to three hours caused by the wait time between procedures. A general sense of dizziness and nausea followed each visit lasting for two days and then gradually faded away. From the time we started on April 30th, every Monday, things went smoothly until June 11th when my blood count was too low for treatment. The doctor skipped the treatment on the 11th doing nothing and on the 18th we resumed the treatments—now using revised medication dosage. All went well until

August 25th when I went to emergency room with high fever and chest pain. I was diagnosed with blood clot in right lung and a low-grade infection. I spent four days in hospital having no chemo treatment that week. Although the hospital called it a chest pain, the clot on my lung made it hurt on my right side and breathing was difficult. I started a new regimen—two weeks of twice daily shots to thin my blood, followed by blood thinner pills. Chemo was restarted Sept 4th and ended on September 24th. During September I had an appointment with the Radiation doctor to set up the radiation treatments, to be given in Green Valley. Treatments started on October 8th and continued five times a week, ending November 9th, 2012. The final hi-intensity radiation treatments were given from November 12th to 20th. The port was removed from my chest on Friday, December 21st, 2012. My second cancer treatment is now complete. I will be on blood-thinner pills for the rest of my life.

This essay was written as a clinical reminder to people who have recently been diagnosed with breast cancer or have found a lump and wonder what will happen to them. After all is said and done, it was my experience that the doctors, nurses, technicians and everyone I came in contact with during my treatments were kind, friendly and compassionate people. To those who presently have the symptoms of cancer, do not despair. You can beat it. So much is being done to eradicate the problem right now and more research is happening daily, that will one day stamp out cancer and kill it forever.

May good fortune be yours.

Chapter Eleven

Shelly Bentz

For me, the most difficult part of my experience with breast cancer was before I was diagnosed. In the fall of 1997 I found a lump in my breast while doing a self-exam. I wasn't too worried about it but knew I was overdue for a mammogram, so I scheduled an appointment. I expected it would take about half an hour or less as it had before, so scheduled it first thing in the morning, planning to go on to work right afterwards. However, this time was different; I spent several hours at the hospital, repeating tests, waiting for a radiologist to read it, and then trying to get a clearer picture of a specific area. It was not the area where I noticed the lump, but was on my other breast. Despite spending most of the day there, I don't recall being told much of anything other than the lump I felt was a fibrous cyst and there was another "suspicious area" which needed further examination.

An appointment was made for me to see a local specialist and I saw him a couple days later. By this time I was very worried about it, but got no answers at all. It was a brief appointment and I don't recall anything was said except he wanted me to see an oncologist who would be there the following day, and they would schedule an appointment for me. When he left the room, I thought he was coming back. Then the nurse came in to tell me I could leave; I asked her questions, but she couldn't tell me anything. I knew what an oncologist was and knew then I must have cancer; I thought it must be bad, pretty far advanced, so they were leaving it to the oncologist to tell me. Despite conscious efforts to keep my imagination under control and not allow my thoughts to "go there," I imagined the worst, and it was one of the worst nights of my life. My family history includes many cases of cancer, including grandparents, an aunt and an uncle. I couldn't help feeling scared of what the future might hold. My husband and I talked about it later, I cried and we prayed.

I saw the oncologist the following day and was told I had Ductal Carcinoma in Situ (DCIS). He explained it was detected early, was a small area and was encapsulated within that area, and removing that section of my breast was recommended. Since this was before "Google," a wonderful friend got out a huge medical reference book on cancer later that day and looked up the diagnosis. That was the most helpful and reassuring information I got. Based on the information she found, she told me, "If you're going to have cancer, this is probably the best kind to have."

I had other tests and biopsies, and the surgery was scheduled within a few days. I felt I needed to tell my children, ages 10 and 13, before the surgery. I don't remember much of what was said but do recall my son, 13, said he had just one question, looked me straight in the eye and asked, "Can it be cured?" I was not prepared for this straight forward question; I reassured him with much more confidence than I felt, told him I would have surgery, some treatment and everything would be just fine. At that time I don't think I could have told him anything else even if it had been a much more serious prognosis. I needed to be able to give him the hope and reassurance that I would be all right and nothing was going to change. This is one aspect that still bothers me and causes me to become emotional when I think about it. Thankfully, I could reassure him with information I had been given, even though I may not have felt all that certain about it myself yet. For an adult, to deal with and accept a diagnosis of breast cancer may be difficult and take some time. It is going to cause some changes. But one of the most difficult parts is how to tell those we love and who love us, especially children, and how to help them deal with it in a beneficial and healthy way.

What I had told my son, although I was very unsure at the time, turned out to be quite accurate. I had a partial mastectomy and radiation therapy was recommended, more as a precautionary measure, I was told. I had six weeks of radiation treatment with no significant problems. I was so thankful for the Carson Radiation Center at Faith Regional Health Services in Norfolk, the wonderful staff there and the knowledge, skill and personable approach of my radiation oncologist. I continued to work at my job full time, taking time each day to go for treatment, and missed only a couple days of work near the end of my treatment because of feeling very tired.

Initially, it seemed as though I remembered every detail, when this happened or when that occurred, the sequence of events and how it affected me. I felt like I would always remember it all, it would always stand out, but as time goes on, the details begin to blur together and fade. Specific aspects of the illness or treatment don't stand out as being so significant. This is a good thing; life goes on, the details are not that important anymore, not such a priority, and can be relegated to their proper place in your life and in your memory.

Early in the summer of 2006 I was diagnosed with breast cancer again. It was in my other breast. As I was having a biopsy, again, I was feeling sorry for myself, thinking "I don't want to go through this again!" The diagnosis was the same, Ductal carcinoma in situ. I remembered "If you're going to have cancer, this is probably the best kind to have." The treatment was the same, and after the surgery was done, I felt like the rest was "a piece of cake." I had "been there, done that" and knew basically what to expect. As in many situations, the unknown is so much more difficult to deal with rationally than when we know the facts and what we can realistically expect to happen.

My journey through cancer had positive benefits. It made me much more aware of the importance of life, helped me understand how quickly everything can change, and the importance of making the best use of the time we are given. It was definitely a learning situation with more medical involvement than I ever had before. The second time through I had a huge advantage because of my prior experience and wish I had known the first time what I knew then. Even though mine was only for a very short time, it also gave me a better understanding of living with a chronic illness, how it impacts every aspect of one's life. Managing or treating the illness has to be a factor in every decision and all plans. After I was diagnosed the second time, my husband and I took a trip to Colorado before I started radiation because we knew that would be the only travelling we would do that summer. Dealing with cancer, the treatment and effects on our life also brought us closer in our marriage.

I believe God has a plan for our lives. I know at times it is hard to see, but it is important to look for positive benefits and possibilities from negative situations. Dwelling on the negative can lead to a feeling of loss of control, blaming, and a downward spiral. I do not believe God causes cancer, but He "works for good for those who love Him." Many things happen over which we have no control; often the only thing we can control is our reaction and how we respond to the situation. Having faith and trusting in God doesn't mean everything will be fine or turn out how we want; it is knowing that God is there with us through it all. He knows better than we do how to help us through any situation, and He will be there and help us cope with whatever comes our way.

There have been discussion and changes in the treatment recommended for DCIS in the past few years. With advances in detection and monitoring, surgery and radiation may not be the first choice of treatment, and a "wait and see" approach may be recommended. Whatever your diagnosis and course of treatment, as you go through your journey with cancer, may you look for and find positive benefits and opportunities. May you know that God knows you by name and He understands what you are going through. He will travel your journey with you and can work for good through our hurts and most difficult times.

Chapter Twelve

Lora Johnson

Happiness is a choice…
Growing up, I have always heard that Happiness is a choice… "You wake up each morning, so you have a choice… be miserable and waste your day, or chose to be happy, Thank God, and maybe even help someone else along the way…

My story started in 2002, our baby boy died after 9 months and 27 days; he never came home from the hospital, but we made University Medical Center our second home and Joshua always had my daddy's spirit, and always had a smile for everyone. After a year, my husband and I decided to adopt; it was June 2003; but my breast Hurt! And it was red and hard and very painful. Don't ever let a doctor or nurse tell you cancer doesn't hurt. I was informed that it could have been that time of the month and to wait and see how I felt in several weeks.

Several weeks later put us in July and now the hard lump that was red and painful was the size of my left palm. Now I went to the woman's clinic at the VA hospital, as I am a disabled veteran. Next thing I know I am meeting with the Oncology surgeon and we are discussing my options. My husband, who has been with me through thick and thin, was by my side once again and telling me, we can handle this. With my father's message in my head, I interrupted the surgeon, held my hand out and said, "Hi, I'm Lora. Always come to me with a good joke and Never say Oops or Oh S%^T in the operating room... I might hear you!"

We got along great and so my relationship with these wonderful doctors, surgeons and especially the nursing and pharmacy staff began ☺

I shocked the surgeon and his resident when I told them that "they", my breasts, were fired!! and to get rid of them. We did the normal tests and biopsies, to find out the cancer was in my left breast and in a few of the lymph nodes in my left armpit; and they were going to do a mastectomy. I had the second or right side removed for safety sake. Since I was only 37 years old at this time, they wanted to do the best they could to save what they could, but I said not to worry... They're fired!!! You see, I say they were fired, because the whole time our boy Joshua was in the hospital, I could not provide enough breast milk to sustain him. I felt like a failure, because even the "breast milk Gestapo" said, dear you're done...

In my head, I have this great mind that tries to put things into perspective for me; as with this... Don't worry, they will cut the breasts off and I will return to work in a week. Silly me... Wow, it's been so long ago, but I spent several days in the hospital and took medical disability from work for several long weeks. I didn't lose my attitude and through it all, I asked God to hold me as he stated in "Footprints". I also believe in angels and asked for their love and guidance. I am more spiritual, and I am Jewish. This being said, whomever you turn to in your times of need, I pray that they provide you with solace and guidance to stay strong and keep your attitude and self at peace and happiness.

I stayed away from negative people and refused to listen to family members and friends that were crying or whiny. I told everyone around me to come to me with support and positive attitudes and a good joke. ☺ My husband was my rock and sometimes pissed me off, because he wasn't going to let me give up my spirit or strength. I used the mantra while getting the hard chemo..."Health and Healing" over and over and over again. I thought about chemo as medicine; just as there are diabetics that take needles every day, I took my medicine, but since I am so afraid of needles, I go to the hospital on my day to get treatment and not only do I get to look away while they put the needle in the PORT, (get a port-a-cath, they are a God-send and keeps the Chemo from terrorizing the veins in your arms. ☺ (Oh! And you get to have free food. ☺ Free food is Always good food.)

I have to tell you I have been extremely fortunate in my life; my husband has been extremely important in my life and supportive. He does push me to stay involved and be strong. I have seen a lot of others who give up and I send cards to their loved ones after their passing; I refuse to give up and give in. I work for FlightSafety International, and they are incredibly generous when it comes to family and their employees. My boss, was there for us during my son's time in the hospital, and while I was dealing with this. May he rest in peace, the founder of FlightSafety, Al Ultchi used to come and visit our center and always made a point to come into my office and see how I was doing and if I needed anything. Due to my surgeries, I could not use the muscles in my chest, and it hurt to 3-hole punch documents, so they bought me an electric 3-hole punch. Go figure ☺ again, it comes back to taking care of each other. My boss Rudy Rostash, would drive to my home and pick me up and take me to work, even if it were for 2 hours and then if I started getting tired, he would drive me home. Not because they wanted me at work, but so that I would not stay home and dwell on my situation. It was extremely therapeutic and I would recommend it to anyone – do not give up your life, keep going. And keep smiling. My niece used to call me from the nurses office almost every day to see how I was doing. She was my cheering section. My family and friends actively stayed in my life and provided me with love and support. My mom would use relaxation techniques on me and teach me how to breathe. My God-mom would stay at the hospital with my husband, to provide him with support, while I was going through surgeries.

Because I am an identical mirror twin, I did the BRACA gene tests, which thank God, I am negative, so no one else in the family has to worry. When I got scared, my husband David would put his head against mine and say we will get through this. We have always had rescued dogs, and he would say that they need me too. ☺ David would give me the white blood cell shots and hold me when I was sick. That Red chemo – YUCK!!! Then I would be so weak, that I got shingles. Wholly Cow!!! But there is a salve called: Acyclovir ointment for shingles.

Miracle Mouth wash or Compound 99 – which contains the following:

Lidocaine, Benadryl, and can contain nystatin, or Maalox.

It was numbing, anti-itch, and either antifungal, or indigestion and soothing relief.

I get asked what meds I was put on. I am a 3 time cancer survivor – Yeah!!!

The fact that I am a survivor is a Yeah moment.

I do remember that one of the drugs was Red and made me really sick. It also made me lose my hair after the first use. I remember waking up, and finding my hair on my pillow. Before I could cry, my husband said, "Quick, get a baggie... we'll bag up your hair and give it to your boss as a joke". ☺ He wasn't too impressed when I gave it to him though; as he is bald and I said I'll get the glue! ☺ heheh. Actually, he had a good sense of humor.

My friend at the American Cancer society, whom I volunteer for, told me it was my turn to get the help, so I met with them and learned about the Giving Closet, where I received a free wig, some scarves and a hat to put on my bald head. I also learned about Look Good, Feel Better, where a cosmetologist gave a seminar on how to color in eye brows, what moisturizers actually worked and how to apply make-up. You really do not realize how important your eye lashes, hairs in your ears and nose hairs are until you lose them and you can't stop the dirt and dust from blowing in your eyes, the sound of gobblety gook instead of words in your ears and the constant dripping... enough said?

I will tell you that if you are losing your hair and your head hurts from Chemo, go to any beauty supply shop and ask for "DooGrow". It's in the African

American section for hair care. It all-natural, calms the scalp, and does promote hair growth.

Recently a dear friend bought me "The Bosley Treatment for Hair", it did help me to grow my hair back full and beautiful, but it does make your skin tingle, so I would not recommend it for when you first start or till you are done with chemo so that you can tolerate this feeling. ☺ I do love these products.

I have been asked how treatment has affected me. When I got the call, actually the doctor was trying to reach my husband; his number is one off from mine. I got the oh-oh feeling, and I have always trusted my feelings; so when she called, I told her, I have cancer? And then fell to the chair in the main entrance area at work. She said that she needed to speak with David and I pretty much forced her hand; I was shaking and falling apart. I asked her. Can I live, Can I live?? She said yes, but it will be a hard road. I said that was fine, but that I could still live right? She said yes, and right then and there I decided to treat this very matter of fact in that I was going to live. That this was just another name for the Flu or Diabetes and they can live through and with it, so I can too!!! I got my direct boss out of a meeting and asked him to sit with me till David could come to get me. Of course he would be with me and he hugged me and both he and his wife would stand beside us for whatever we needed. I was on so many prayer wheels and chains.

I personally had other issues that I was dealing with. We were still dealing with the loss of our son, our fathers, both of them, had passed away, along with David's Godfather. Then our son died. Then one of our dogs decided to up and die, I think to be with Joshua. It was a very, very sad time in our lives, but we always knew that we had to be strong for each other, our surviving dogs and other family members.

So in closing stay strong, with the Belief in your God. Stay happy. Keep a positive attitude and don't let this get you down. You can live with cancer.

Chapter Thirteen

Claudie Wilson

I'm in a straightjacket. That was my first thought as my eyes cracked open the morning after my mastectomy. Then, as consciousness seeped in, I found that I could move my arms a bit. It was only my torso that was tightly bound

The year was 1986, and it was the beginning of what would prove to be a long recovery from breast cancer. The cancer had been caught early and my surgeon told me I was fortunate. Each of the eight lymph nodes harvested had tested benign. My breast was gone, but the cancer hadn't spread.

Five more days would pass before the bandages came off and I saw what my chest looked like. During that time I underwent physical therapy and learned arm stretches to combat lymphedema – a common side effect of a mastectomy, when the lymph nodes are removed and their drainage function disrupted. One stretch consisted of walking my fingers up a wall, from waist level to as far above my head as I could reach. In those first post-op days, shoulder height was as high as I could manage, and it felt as if the skin under my arm would rip open. I was encouraged to grit my teeth and persevere, to keep my shoulder joint loose and regain my range of motion, in order to combat lymph fluid buildup in my arm.

I was given a Teddy Bear to hug when I had to cough or sneeze – To clasp the bear tightly to my chest so that the sudden lung expansion wouldn't pop my stitches. A Reach to Recovery volunteer visited me in my hospital room and brought post-mastectomy bras to show me. This American Cancer Society program is dedicated to improving the quality of life for breast cancer patients, survivors, and their families. The advocates are usually breast cancer survivors themselves, and can be an invaluable resource for information, comfort and understanding.

The evening before I was scheduled to be discharged, my surgeon came to remove the bandages. He also removed. the drain lines he'd stitched under my skin to control excess fluid. When the gauze was unwound and lay in a pink-tinged pile on my blanket, I finally looked down on myself. The normal breast was creased and discolored, but intact. On the other side of my chest, the skin lay flat against my ribs, bisected diagonally by an eight-inch, red incision line.

My doctor gave me a morphine injection and went to work snipping and tugging to pull out the rubber tubing of the drains. The morphine made me vomit, but did little to alleviate the physical pain. What it did accomplish was to dull, temporarily at least, the emotional shock of my new appearance.

I was 33 years old and reconstruction was a given. My plastic surgeon had decided on a 2-stage procedure using a temporary tissue expander, which had been inserted immediately after my breast was removed. It's essentially a flat-backed empty implant with a port through which saline is injected through the skin on a regular schedule until it's gradually inflated to the desired size. Then it is swapped out for a permanent implant. After a month's recovery time, my incision and surgical site were sufficiently healed to begin the inflation process, which would take six months. And, lucky for me, so many nerves had been cut during the mastectomy that I didn't feel the needles used to inject saline into the expander. I had little discomfort in the area other than a feeling of tightness as the skin over the expander was progressively strtched to accommodate its growing size. Once the desired volume was reached, the exchange was performed on an outpatient basis at the same hospital where I'd had the mastectomy. I was relieved and elated. The painful experience of breast cancer was behind me. I could now forget about it and get back to my normal life.

As the years passed, my body changed, as all bodies do when approaching middle age. I gained some weight and became softer and rounder. I'd been skinny all my life, so it was a welcomed progression. But I soon found myself dealing daily with the simple logistics of an artificial bosom. Devoid of normal fatty tissue, my re-engineered breast didn't grow like my normal breast did. Dressing to maintain a symmetrical appearance became an increasing challenge. After ten years had passed I began wearing silicone breast prosthesis to even things out. It was a constant reminder of my disease.

Another issue arose twenty-two years after my mastectomy. I was reading a magazine in the dentist's office when I came across an article about breast implants. It stated that their lifespan was ten to twenty years, depending on their composition and placement in the body (under the muscle tissue or on top of it). After that time they were prone to rupture, or "fail", as the article termed it. Concerned, I contacted my plastic surgeon. Since in the ensuing years I'd moved across the country, I was advised to consult a local physician immediately. When the new doctor examined me, she confirmed that my implant was past due for failure, and needed to be replaced with a new one right away.

That operation would not require a hospital admission. The old implant was removed and exchanged for a new silicone version as an outpatient procedure and I would be allowed to recuperate at home. Within two days my entire upper chest was dark purple. My doctor diagnosed a hematoma, presumably caused by internal bleeding at the surgical site. The new implant was contaminated and would have to be removed without delay in order to avoid infection and further complications. I was rushed back to surgery where a quart of blood and fluid was cleared from my chest. The old implant was replaced with a new one. It was over and I was released from my physician's care. This was final. I was done.

As I healed and the new implant settled into place, it began to gradually shift toward the center of my chest. Soon I had no demarcation between where one breast ended and the other began. I tried to reach my physician without success. I drove to her office and found the place locked up and a sign on the door that announced she had closed her practice. Another setback.

I found a new plastic surgeon and, when he examined me, he decided that the best course of action was to start over – remove the implant, let my chest heal, and begin again with a saline tissue expander. I was mentally jerked back to 1986.

This time the inflation process was familiar and went smoothly. Three months after the tissue expander was situated and gradually inflated with saline, it had reached desirable size and was replaced with a permanent silicone implant. My chest was back to normal for the third and final time.

I never experienced the mourning of a lost body part, as some mastectomy patients do. What the experience brought to me was a new perspective on the impermanence of life. The little things we all take for granted - good health, planning into the future, simply getting dressed every day- shifted to a new reality. I endured the diagnosis and the many surgeries because I had to. I wasn't "strong", as some people called me. That implies choice, and there are precious few choices associated with cancer. You can't just say "I won't do it." You have to do it.

I got through it because it was the hand I was dealt, and part of my destiny.

I got through it because I'm a survivor.

Chapter Fourteen

Pam

On December 9, 2009, I asked about a lump under my right arm while at my regular doctor's appointment. On Labor Day weekend, I had the flu and it puffed up to the size of a marble. Then I got my flu shot in October and it puffed up again. My doctor sent me to a surgeon since it had changed. I got in to see the surgeon on December 17th at 9:00. They set up a CT-scan and a mammogram at the local hospital's radiology department for 3:30 that afternoon. By the time I arrived, they had changed the order to include an ultrasound. Everything indicated a cyst and I went back to the surgeon to have it drained on December 21st. When the surgeon tried to drain it, it was solid, so I wound up having a needle biopsy. I was supposed to get the results on December 30th, but the surgeon was out of town, so they said they would call me with the results. Instead they told me to come in Monday, January 4th, 2010, at 3:30 to discuss the results.

I worried all weekend since they asked me to come in. It was breast cancer. They set up a modified radical mastectomy for January 11th and a CT-scan for 4:30 on January 6th. I worked at the Madison County Courthouse, which closed at 2:30 that day due to the weather. Once I had returned to Norfolk, I went straight to the hospital and they got me in in a short time.

I had to be at the hospital by 5:30 a.m. on January 11th. My sister, Gail, stayed overnight after she and her husband came to town for Sunday Church. She took me to the hospital in the morning. My sister-in-law, BJ, arrived about 6 am. They told me after the anesthetist gave me something in my IV, I sounded drunk and I said "I feel drunk," but I don't remember saying that.

I went to surgery about 7:25 and I was out of surgery about 9:00. I woke up about 9:30, but everything was quite hazy, and by 10:00, I was taken to my room. BJ stayed until 4:30 and Gail stayed until 9 that night. I didn't have a good night. My back hurt and it didn't help to raise or lower the head of the bed. Then about 2:30 am my kidneys decided to get rid of all the fluids they had administered to me.

I was released about noon Tuesday, January 12th. I had two drains with bulbs that I called big, fat ticks that I named Curly and Larry. I had to drain them twice a day.

I went back to the surgeon on Monday, January 18th. I got rid of Curly on that day, but Larry was still draining too much. The lump was a 4 cm tumor and of the 12 lymph nodes that were removed, one, the size of 1.1 cm, tested positive for cancer. The rest were clear. Gail stayed with me until after my appointment with the surgeon. What a blessing to have a sister who cares enough to do that. My first visit with the oncologist was set for February 2nd.

January 20, 2010: I seem to always be waiting for something. A part of me says "I hope, I hope, there is no need for chemo", but another part of me says "let's not take any chances and zap any tiny bits of cancer which may be hiding." I'll cross that bridge when I get there. The First bridge – biopsy, Second bridge – diagnosis, Third bridge – surgery, Fourth bridge – getting rid of Curly. Next - Larry must go.

When I awoke from surgery, most of my chest was numb, along with the back of my upper arm. As the feeling started returning, I ache and my armpit feels raw. My breastbone hurt from the start. The surgeon said they scrape the attachments off the breastbone so that will be sore for a while. I should get back the feeling in my arm within a couple months.

January 21, 2010: Larry is gone! The second drain came out today. When the drainage decreased, it did so in a hurry. It appears my incision is healing very well. The area under the arm feels raw. It is in a fold and it is very hard to keep dry. The surgeon said to try to keep the 4X4 gauze pads in that area so it can finish healing. Now I wait for the visit to the oncologist.

My cousin, Connie, wrote. For some reason she decided that I must be very brave. She said that Aunt Dena is smiling down on me from Heaven. Aunt Dena was diagnosed with breast cancer in the 1970s at about the same age as I was, and with a tumor in the same place. She felt it while taking a shower and had a mastectomy. Accepting reality and moving on about covers it. I think I learned that from my maternal grandmother and probably from my mother and her sisters, Dena and Vera. Come to think of it, they all are probably smiling down at me from Heaven and praying for me.

My grandmother arranged a rosary for me, and I am on seven prayer chains at various churches. When I added all the other individuals who are praying for me, I am impressed.

January 22, 2010: I sometimes wonder why I am not freaking. Is it a defense mechanism, or is it that I have accepted that I have breast cancer and I am simply moving on. The strongest emotion I seem to have is a warm fuzzy feeling, realizing how much people do care about me. The hardest part is the waiting; for the pain to leave, for the chemo to begin, and hopefully I will do okay with that. It is very frustrating that except for the right arm and chest, I feel good, but I can't do much. I just have to be patient. The doctor wants me to walk around, but when it comes to shopping, my brother, Doug, who lives with me, has to push the cart and lift anything that requires two hands. He isn't too happy about that.

January 23, 2010: Doug is sick. He had a bit of a temperature last night and aches today. I hope he doesn't give it to me. I'll have to go pick up a few things from the grocery store later. I had a strange dream last night that the surgeon's office wanted me to pay them $6,400.00. Since that is beyond the stop-loss on my insurance policy, so I don't need to worry about that. I just need to figure out how to come up with an extra $2,300.00.

I picked up a few items from the grocery store that we were running out of. I had to pull the cart since I couldn't push it. It is amazing how people were so willing to help. When I got home, I have to take a long nap as I still get tired so easily.

There are quite a few areas of the incision where the surface has healed. I'm trying to do the exercise where I walk my fingers up a wall a couple times a day. The rest of the movement is pretty much coming naturally, since I am right-handed and my right side is affected, but reaching up needs some work.

I'm hoping that another two weeks brings a reduction in the pain so I can go back to work.

Other than the right chest and arm, and the fact that I get so tired so easily, the rest of me feels fine. It can be so frustrating when I see something I want to do but I can't. It will come I guess. I just need to be patient. My niece, Tammy, had a great idea when she sent me this journal.

January 24, 2010: I wonder how soon I will be able to get my prosthesis. I keep catching myself sitting crooked by leaning to the left. Is my remaining breast heavy enough to pull me that far off balance? I told Gail, "Just think how frustrated I would be if it were warm enough to hang clothes out and I couldn't do it."

January 25, 2010: It's been cold and windy. What do I expect? It's January in Nebraska. I need to mail the paperwork to my brother, Al, so he can figure my income tax, so that I can pay some bills. The bills just keep coming. That's what worries me the most.

January 27, 2010: I balanced my checkbook and then spent an hour trying to figure out what I owe on medical bills. With the buy down on the insurance deductible and my 125 Flex Plan and medical bills from all directions, it is confusing. I keep compiling them. I still haven't seen the bill from my surgery, just pathology, CT-scans, mammograms, ultrasounds, doctors' office visits, etc.

January 28, 2010: I meet with the oncologist on February 2nd. May be I'll find out what stage we are talking about. I'm hoping for stage I. I hope the incision will be healed by then so I can start chemo. I'm getting impatient for healing and to get started on the next step. I am concerned with the fatigue and nausea as side effects and also chemo brain. Hair loss I can deal with. I don't know how many nasty side effects I will have. It would be nice to know what side effects I can expect and how long the chemo lasts. The year stared out horribly. Hopefully it will end great.

February 1, 2010: Tomorrow I find out what's next. I need to be at the Carson Cancer Center for lab work at 8:00 am and presumably to talk with the oncologist. Chemo will have to wait until I heal a little more. On Thursday, January 28th, the scab came off the area just outside my armpit. It looked pretty good Friday, then about midnight it started hurting. When I checked it, it looked like the incision might be opening up. Well, the skin was.

I got in to see a doctor on Saturday. She put me on antibiotics and said I was to see her, my primary care physician or my surgeon on Monday – today. Then Saturday night at bedtime, I got out my chair and felt something pop under my arm. I then felt a glugging under my arm. I realized there was a lot of swelling under my arm and I was sloshing. By Sunday morning it seemed a little better and by this morning was quite a bit better.

I got in to see the surgeon at 2:45 pm. He walked into the waiting room and said, "Pam, come on you trouble maker." He was teasing me as usual. He thought the incision, which had opened up, didn't look too bad. I am to use triple antibiotic cream on the open area only. He also checked my shoulder blade which had been fairly solid and swollen. I hadn't thought too much about that. I figured it was just because of the surgery and that the numbness would disappear when the swelling went down. Well it did in a hurry after I started sloshing. That was probably where the fluid came from. By now it is pretty well gone. Of course, now my shoulder feels raw as the feeling returns.

I have resorted to writing on a calendar. The antibiotics are every six hours and the Tylenol is every eight hours. To make sure I remember which one I took when is why I write it down.

February 2, 2010: I am at the oncologist's. Maybe now I'll know where I stand as far as the prognosis. I still don't know Stage or anything else about the cancer. It would be nice to know, I think.

The tumor tested HER2 Positive (2%). We are doing four cycles of chemo. My next appointment is in one week. Meanwhile I will have a MUGA scan to check my heart function on Thursday and an ultrasound scan of the liver to check a .9 cm spot on my liver. If the ultrasound of the liver is okay, then I am early Stage II.

On Friday I have surgery to insert a port for the chemo. I need to be at the hospital at 7:15 am. Gail? BJ? One of you will get to take me.

I have to admit I am a bit worried. If the ultrasound shows any indication of cancer, everything changes. It's one step forward, and wait, and so on.

February 3, 2010: Tomorrow is the MUGA scan and ultrasound. Hopefully everything comes back okay and the part of the incision that opened up will heal quickly so that we can get going on chemo. I guess I am just impatient to get on with my life and get this over with, It gets so frustrating with wanting to get back to normal and do things like I used to but not being able to.

I have to use the right arm as much as I can but I have to be careful not to overdo it since it's the right arm and I am right handed. I keep doing more that I should and then I wind up hurting. It's a very fine balancing act.

I keep wondering if the chemo will make my hair fall out. Some chemo drugs do and some don't. It's no big deal if it does, but I'd like to know if I need to get a wig and should I get my hair shaved.

February 4, 2010: Well the ultrasound and the MUGA scan are done. The ultrasound tech had a lot of trouble finding the questionable area on the liver. She said it was like looking for a needle in a haystack. It was vague on the CT-scan.

For the MUGA scan, they drew a syringe of my blood and mixed it with the radioactive whatever and after 25 minutes, re-inject it into the vein. Then they take two pictures each taking 10 minutes. They change the angle of the scanner between the scans. Hopefully everything comes back good.

Tomorrow it's time for the port. I am hoping that the fact that the spot on the liver was indistinct on the CT-scan and difficult to find is good news, and there are no, or at least minimal cardiac problems.

The hospital outpatient surgery center just called and delayed the time I need to be there until 9:00 A.M., which will be better for BJ. She doesn't have to take me so early.

February 8, 2010: The hospital called again and delayed the time to 10:30 A.M. After I got there it only took a couple minutes to register. No more than I got to sit down, they took me back to pre-op. They gave me Celebrex and Vicodin before surgery to control pain. After they inserted the IV it seemed like no time at all and I was on my way to the operating room. It didn't take long to hook the monitors. The next thing I knew, I was waking up. The procedure was done. I did find an EKG sticky patch on my back yesterday. After the mastectomy, Gail found another one.

I think I had more pain on the right side even though the port is on the left side. The port side is still very tender. I never filled the prescription for pain killers, but I have been getting by with Tylenol. Tomorrow, I go back to the oncologist. I hope it is good news.

Gail asked me to go with her Thursday to her pain doctor for her shots in the neck since she can't drive after getting them. Finally, something I can do something to help her. She has been great helping me with housework. I do what I can to help her with it, but there is only so much I can do.

Yesterday I hurt quite a bit. Today seems to be much better. May be I am turning the corner. The open area on the suture line hasn't closed yet. It seems to be filling in from underneath and now from the side.

February 9, 2010: Well, I'm waiting at the oncologist's office. I'm trying not to worry too much about the test results, but it is kind of hard not to be concerned. There are a couple of things that I need to remember to ask about. Do I need to continue taking the antibiotics? What possible side effects can I expect? What is a cycle? I will probably have to check my blood sugar more often just to make sure it stays where it should be. I admit I don't check it as often as I should. I also need to take the "dressing" off the incision for the port. It looks like a piece of plastic wrap.

A cycle is one day every three weeks. I need to continue the antibiotics for another five days. I am early Stage IIA, according to the oncologist. I may or may not lose my hair, but the other possible side effects should be easier to control. I go back next Tuesday to see if the incision is healed well enough to start chemo on Wednesday.

Thursday I am going along with Gail to Columbus for her appointment with her pain doctor so I can drive her back. Yesterday and today the pain is much less. Maybe by next week I can go back to work. There just isn't much on TV that I want to watch and that I haven't already seen.

February 11, 2010: One month ago today I had my mastectomy and I am still not completely healed along the incision. About 9:00 a.m. Gail and I left for Columbus. I forgot to take my antibiotic before I left and we didn't get back until about 4:00 P.M., so I was an hour late for the next dose.

February 16, 2010: I went to see the surgeon yesterday. He thought the incision that had opened up looked good and is now very superficial, but healed well enough to start chemo. The oncologist looked at it this morning and agreed, so I start chemo tomorrow. I asked how likely it will be that I am going to lose my hair. He said about a 70% chance, so I went to the resource center and asked about getting a free wig.

They had a real nice one in a style and color that I liked and that looked good on me, so I took it. Then on the way home, I stopped at my hair dresser's because I definitely needed a haircut and since I have the wig, I decided to get it cut really short. My hair dresser used the clipper and trimmed it to about a half an inch. I wore the wig home. I dug out some scarves to see if I can use them at home so I don't have to wear the wig all the time.

The oncologist said that the 9mm spot on the liver is probably not anything to worry about, but after finishing chemo, we will do another CT-scan to make sure it hasn't changed. Then I will start hormone therapy with Aromasin, which has fewer side effects and is for women who are postmenopausal.

The surgeon agreed that I could try to start back to work. He said to start with two hours and work up to full days, which is good since it has been only five weeks and he said it would take eight to ten weeks before I could go back. He said on the day of chemo and the day after, I would probably be wiped out. Well, that would only be two days times four, which would be a total of eight days. If I can get back to work soon I will still have some sick leave. I am concerned about nausea and the possibility of fatigue. As for hair loss, I have a wig and my hair will grow back. I'm hoping when it does, it will come back curlier. My oncologist said sometimes it comes back twice as curly. That would be nice.

I think I will need to get blood work done weekly and see the oncologist every third week. I'll have to check tomorrow. I will also have to make sure Gail will be able to take me tomorrow. They want someone to bring you the first time to make sure you will be okay driving afterwards. I need to be there at 8:30. If Gail can't take me, then I have a couple other people who probably can help out.

February 17, 2010: I had chemo today; first I had to start taking the Dexamethasone twice a day yesterday, today and tomorrow. This morning when I went in, first they flushed the port. Then I got Benadryl and more flushing the port again. Next it was Docetaxel which took one and a half hours. They give it slowly to make sure I didn't have an adverse reaction. The port was flushed once more, followed by Cyclophosefamide, which took an hour. It was 12:30 when I got done. After the chemo they had to (what else), flush the port with saline and re-prime it with Herceptin.

So far, I'm doing okay. If I'm okay tomorrow, I will call my boss and try going in for a half a day to see how it goes. They will probably appreciate the help. I should feel bad about being gone for almost six weeks, but it has been a rough five and a half weeks. Hopefully I'm going to be up to it. I have recovered enough that I need to be able to do something. We will see how I feel in the morning.

I will need to get my shot of Neulasta to help the bone marrow produce more white blood cells, so I'm not too vulnerable to infection. I need to go in at 1:00, so maybe I'll try 8:30 to 12:30 tomorrow. We will just have to see how I feel in the morning.

February 18, 2010: When I woke up at 6:45 this morning, I felt good, so I got up, fed the cats and ate some breakfast. I called my boss then. I had been calling ever so often to keep her up to date as to how I was doing. She was happy that everything went so well with the chemo. When I asked about coming in for half the day until 12:30, she said they would be happy to see me.

I was getting a little bit tired by 11:00, but it really felt good to be back at work even if it was only for half a day. Everyone was glad to see me and asked how I was doing. My friend, Linda's daughter, Tara, is having a double mastectomy Wednesday, February 24th. A friend gave me Tara's address so I can write to her. She doesn't know me from Jane Doe, but maybe I can be of some support for her since I've been there, done that. At her age it is probably much more distressing than it is for me. I hope I can find the right words to encourage her.

February 19, 2010: It is the second day back at work. It seems to be working out for me to go in and work until 12:30 p.m. I figure that is when I would normally go to lunch and it is only half an hour more than half a day. I have to take a nap when I get home, but at least I am getting out and starting to get back to something resembling normal. A friend of mine, Nancy, asked if I wanted to go to our favorite restaurant, Burrito King, for lunch. I needed to eat something, so I went. She wanted to know how I was doing. I also told her about the letter I sent Tara, as she also knows Tara's mother, Linda.

Tara is so young to have breast cancer. She is only 31, I hope what I wrote is in some way helpful. If nothing else, if she tells Linda about it, Linda will appreciate it. This could be much harder on Linda, emotionally, than it is on Tara. I know that my cancer is much harder on my sister Gail than it is on me.

I have accepted it and I'm moving on. I'm optimistic about the outcome. I will beat this. I think when I told Gail, she immediately thought of losing her beloved Daddy to cancer and now she fears losing her big sister. Well she isn't getting rid of me. I'm going to outlive her! As I put in the post script to Tara. Keeping this journal helps deal with the frustration of what I can't do – like work a full day.

I gave my boss a copy of the doctor appointments and I am keeping a bit of time in and out separately, rather than on the regular calendar, so it won't take up all the room on the calendar.

February 20, 2010, Saturday: I didn't breeze through the chemo quite as well as I first thought. My chemo started on Ash Wednesday, February 17th. That day I had a number of hot flashes. On Thursday, I got my Neulasta shot at 1:00 and went home to take a two hour nap. By bedtime, I knew I was getting a bit constipated. Other than that, I felt fine, so I went in again. I did have a fit of heartburn a couple times Friday morning, which wasn't all that bad. On the way home, I started feeling achy. After stopping at the store to pick up a few things, I went home for a two hour nap. I didn't quite finish my lunch and when it came to supper, I ate very little. I just wasn't hungry. Other than that, I felt pretty good.

At 2:00 A.M. I woke up with a gut ache. After eating some yogurt, I was able to doze off again. I really didn't feel the best this morning, but I went to our regular Saturday morning breakfast with my brother, Doug. I didn't finish it all.

We got the groceries and a few other things and got home by 10:30. I went back to bed at 11:00 and slept until 2:00. I then laid there until 5:00 aching. I got up and had a half glass of milk and a piece of dry toast. I did feel a little better after that. I have to admit that I am wondering if what I am going through is typical, or if I am reacting strangely. Is there anything I can do to minimize the reactions for the next cycle. I need to be at work as much as I can or I will run out of sick leave. I do have four weeks of vacation yet, and almost seven weeks of sick leave, but I don't want to wipe it all out.

February 21, 2010: Today seems better. I was able to eat breakfast. I'm still tired but I did sleep fairly well. At 2:00 a.m., I was up for about half an hour and had a little milk. At least the smell of Doug's bacon didn't bother me. I also started a loaf of bread in the bread machine. Hopefully, I will be able to go to work tomorrow. Time will tell. As much as I have been sleeping, I'm guessing it is fatigue.

I am able to eat today as long as I don't try to eat too much. If I don't feel better tomorrow, I don't know if I will be able to go to work. My joints ache, my teeth ache and my feet tingle every so often.

February 22, 2010: I made it to 12:30 today. I wasn't sure I would because my back was hurting. I don't know if it was the chemo, the Neulasta or from spending most of Saturday in bed sleeping. I seem to be suffering from fatigue as well as a very sore back, but at least my food tastes right again. I'm not eating half as much as I used to, which means I'm eating correct amounts instead of pigging out.

Linda was at another office to work this morning. I talked to her for a few minutes. I told her I had sent Tara a letter and hoped it would give her something good to hold on to. At least it made Linda feel good. Sometimes it is the family members who are the most stressed. They can only do so much and feel helpless that they can't do more.

February 23, 2010: I had my blood drawn on my way home. I'm going to ask about talking to the dietician in two weeks when I go in. Also, how can I head off the worst symptoms on the next cycle. It sure would be nice to sleep through the night.

Yesterday, I would have loved to have one of Gail's ambient and a muscle relaxant. If I lay in bed too long, my back hurts. I can't sleep on my back and have been told not to sleep on my right side. That doesn't give me very many options. If I sit in the recliner too long, my butt hurts.

I hate to live on Tylenol. I try not to take more than one or two doses of the arthritis strength, but a lot of days I need a third dose to dull the discomfort.

February 24, 2010: I feel better today. Of course, it probably helped that I actually slept six straight hours for the first time since the mastectomy. I first fell asleep about 10:00 p.m. I woke up about midnight and went to the bathroom. I settled down and the next thing I knew, it was 6:00 a.m. My back feels alot better today.

If I am going to hurt that bad from the Neulasta from day two through day six, that will be tough. Of course, there are only three more cycles. I may be lucky and the rest won't be so bad. We'll just have to take it one cycle at a time.

At last, one cycle down and three more to go. I am hoping that I won't need additional chemo ever, but if I do, I'll do what I need to do. I still can't make it past 12:30 at work. I'm hoping to be able to increase the time at work, maybe next week. Maybe if I get exercise, I will overcome the tiredness.

February 25, 2010: I didn't sleep very well last night. I kept thinking about Tara and remembering my night in the hospital. Finally, about 1:00 a.m., I decided this is the pits. I hardly slept that first night and thought that doesn't mean Tara isn't. I hoped it was "sympathetic insomnia". Just like that, I fell asleep and didn't wake up until 6:00 a.m.

I told my boss that tomorrow I am going to bring my lunch and eat it there. If an hour break and relaxing gives me a little bit of second wind to work a little longer, that will be good. I won't know if I don't try it.

Linda emailed Nancy, who passed it on to me. Tara went into surgery at 1:00 p.m. yesterday and got out at 6:00 p.m. She was having nausea problems, but after five hours for the double mastectomy and reconstruction, she would be nauseous and groggy. Hopefully, they were able to find the right meds to take care of that.

Nancy said that Vaughn and Linda are going to be there for a couple of weeks. That will be a great help for Tara. She will need help with things like housework for another month. Of course if it is just her, no pets, etc., and a dishwasher, that will help.

February 26, 2010: I made it to about 2:45 today. I needed a nap when I got home, but at least it is a step in the right direction. Almost 6 hours, only a little over two more hours to go. I wonder if I can get up to full days before the next cycle.

A customer asked me if I was wearing a wig. She realized I must be a cancer patient. It takes one to spot one. She just passed her five year anniversary. She had eight cycles to my 4 cycles, so she thinks I must be doing okay.

I don't think I will be back to choir until after chemo. The chemo makes my throat a bit raw and I don't want to risk damaging my voice by singing now and not being able to sing later.

February 28, 2010: I made it to church today for the first time since surgery. Many people were surprised to see me and many people stopped me to ask how I am doing. I have never gotten so many hugs in one day. I talked to Cindy, our choir director, to explain why I won't be back to choir this Spring. I have found that when I try singing along with songs on the radio, my throat feels raw. I told Cindy I don't want to try singing now when my throat is so sensitive from the chemo and may not be able to sing later.

Since choir is out, I will go to Sunday school instead. I must admit it is a little bit difficult to not sing during the church service, but I will make a conscious effort to keep my mouth shut.

March 1, 2010: I made it to about 3:50 today. I was tired and didn't get my nap. My niece, Tammy, called me and we talked for a while.

March 3, 2010: Yesterday I made it to about 4:00 before leaving work. If I hadn't needed to have my blood work, maybe I could have stayed longer. Today I did make it to 5:00 – A FULL day at work. I started back half days three weeks and three days after surgery. I was able to do a full day after seven weeks and two days. That's good. Really good considering that my surgeon said I might be able to go back part time in six to eight weeks and it might take 10 weeks.

I am going to have to see how I do next week with cycle two of the chemo. Hopefully I will do okay and not have to miss too much work

March 5, 2010: Last night my scalp hurt so I started rubbing it. I soon realized that part of the reason is I am shedding big time. If I keep this up, I will be bald in a week. Well, it will grow back. With any luck it will grow back thicker and curlier. My eyelashes and eyebrows are getting much more sparse. My legs and arms have very little hair and I haven't had to shave my armpits in two weeks. I also haven't had to shave my chin hairs in a couple weeks.

I wonder how the second cycle of chemo will go next Tuesday. If I follow the pattern of the first cycle. I will feel lousy on Friday. That is not a good day to be wiped out, I have been trying to get to work about 10 minutes early so that I can walk up and down the hall a couple times and get more exercise at home. The first week I didn't eat as much, but this week I have been pigging out.

March 7, 2010: I picked up a prayer shawl for Tara at church today. I will send it to her tomorrow. Thank God that her pathology report came back good. I hope her pain is decreasing. Unfortunately mine got worse as the nerves regenerated. Of course that doesn't mean that Tara's did.

My second cycle is the day after tomorrow. I hope I get by at least as well as I did on the first cycle. It would be nice if I got by better. I need to get a note written to Tara so she knows why she is getting a prayer shawl.

March 8, 2010: Tomorrow is chemo. I must say the Dexamethazone tastes terrible. No wonder you need to take it with food. I'm trying to take it 12 hours apart. I told Gail, that since I did so well on the first cycle that I would be able to drive myself to and from chemo so that she won't need to make an extra trip on Tuesdays. It is very early for a person who doesn't do mornings. Actually, I don't do much better, but I've been getting up early for so long that I just push myself to get going. It has gotten to where it is a bit difficult not to do that.

I went to the post office on my lunch hour and mailed Tara's prayer shawl and get well card. I put a note in it why she was getting a prayer shawl. After I had sealed it, I realized that I started to explain the prayer shawl, I had jumped to her cat, and then back to the prayer shawl. I told her that my shawl went to the hospital for my surgery, to doctors appointments and now to chemo treatments.

I wonder if I will have as many hot flashes. I am hoping to be back full time the rest of the week. I need to remember to take something to eat, as I will probably be late getting lunch tomorrow.

March 9, 2010: I finished cycle two of chemo today about 1:00. My oncologist gave me a prescription for nausea and one for pain to head off the problems I had from the first cycle. I didn't have any hot flashes yet today, but knowing I could, I was careful not to get too warm as that usually starts them. Before I got too warm, I took off my sweater and sat there in the chemo suite in my tank top while everyone else wore sweaters or covered up with blankets.

The steroids make me hyper and the Benadryl makes me groggy. I knew I couldn't go to work.

I am pretty sure my surgeon will okay the prostheses when I go in next Monday. I called the store that handles them and mastectomy bras already and checked with my health insurance to see how many they will pay for. I can get three every 365 days. I also called my dentist to cancel my appointment and I will reschedule after I am done with chemo and my system has a chance to settle down. I will also get my eyes checked in a couple months.

I had to lay down for a couple hours. It was more like a couple of cat naps rather than sleeping, but it did seem to help. Tomorrow I have to get my Neulasta shot, so I will eat a quick lunch, then run back to Norfolk for my shot, and then go back to work. I know what to watch for, so maybe I won't miss much more time this week.

March 11, 2010: I did start hurting from the Neulasta shot today, but Hydrocodone seems to be doing the trick. Yes, I do hurt some, but nothing like I did three weeks ago. I am really tired, but other than that, I seem to be okay. I had a little nausea yesterday, but that was because I wasn't drinking my milk like I usually do.

Tuesday night I was hot. At least last night I slept well. Hopefully, I will tonight. I am starting to be able to taste food again. Last time it took five days, so three days is an improvement. I hope I will be able to get through tomorrow okay, what with it being Friday. If we are busy at work I will probably get really tired.

March 12, 2010: It was a rough day; I found my blood pressure was low. That might explain why I slept all day on Saturday after the first Chemo cycle, since that time corresponds to Friday this time. I will have to check if the drop is typical, or if I have to do something about it. I am really tired. I am thinking of just going to bed. I suppose I need to do the litter boxes. At least Taco John's soft shell and Ole's with Nacho cheese didn't bother my stomach. I have kind of been waiting for 8:30 to take pain killers, but I suppose if I hurt too bad, I can get up and take them later. I just need a nap.

Mary L. Maas

March 13, 2010: I fell asleep on the couch for about an hour, so I got up and did the litter boxes and went to bed. About 1:00 a.m. I got up and took a couple Tylenol. From then I would sleep a couple hours and wake up. I was having strange dreams about different people. I can't remember what they were about, but they involved my brothers and a neighbor. Today I am so tired that I am up for a couple hours, then nap for an hour. I forgot to watch my favorite TV show last night.

I am craving salty or spicy. I can't taste sweet, so maybe that is why I crave salty or spicy.

It was totally beyond me to make it to my cousin's funeral today. I hope her kids understand and I sent a card to explain. I have to remember to set the clocks back tonight. It doesn't seem to be that time of the year yet. Where has winter gone? Next, spring will be gone.

March 15, 2010: I got my prosthesis today. The fitter said many women want as light of prosthesis as possible. Why? If you don't have any weight it is up in the air and you aren't even or balanced.

While doing chemo, I started working on an afghan for Gail's youngest son, Matthew. I did a lot of the work on it at chemo and while I couldn't do much else. When my surgeon walked into the examining room, he asked if I had done all that while waiting. I told him, "Of course."

My prosthesis has enough weight that my bosom is balanced and hopefully my shoulders will be even.

I called Linda yesterday. I wanted to be sure she was coping okay. Mommies want to make it all better for their children, but with breast cancer, the patient has to do what they need to do and their loved ones will just need to love them. There is probably a lot of frustration since all they can do is to be there. They can't fix it. Linda talked for quite a while, which I hope was good for her.

She said Tara is thinking of going back to work after three weeks, which may be pushing it a bit. Tara told Linda and Vaughn she would be alright to be alone after they left Wednesday (March 10). Tara was sort of regretting it. She did tell Linda about the prayer shawl I had sent, which got there after they left. Linda had taken one with her, but she thought the prayer shawl I sent seemed to mean more to Tara. Probably because it was sent by a fellow breast cancer patient and was not something she was expecting. Maybe something in my notes or the prayer shawl has helped Tara. I am pretty sure it helped Linda.

March 23, 2010: Tara sent me a thank you note. That was so sweet of her. It was obvious why the prayer shawl I sent was the one that meant so much to her. It was from someone who is going through the same thing and my notes were notes of encouragement. I told her to not take it too seriously when people always seem to tell you about the worst and don't tell you about all the people who do very well.

I guess I have been lucky in that I keep talking to people who have done well and who have gotten four or five years out from diagnosis. I intend to be around for another 40 years!

I told Gail that since Easter is the Sunday after Chemo, she is welcome to do Easter here for her family. I'm not going to be up to going anywhere. If it doesn't work out for her, Doug can put in a little ham for us.

I am going to ask my oncologist about my blood pressure dropping in the days after chemo. Should I not take my BP meds and should I stay home on Friday? I don't want to miss any more time from work than I have to, but if my blood pressure drops like it did after cycle two and probably did after cycle one, I am not doing anyone any favors.

I seem to be getting over the cold fairly well that I caught. It's a good thing I came down with it this week rather than last week. That could have been bad as my immune system was a lot worse last week. By this week, I have bounced back quite a ways and I seem to be recovering fairly quickly, about like I normally do.

March 28, 2010: Tuesday is chemo cycle number three. After that there is just one more. Hopefully after number four and the CT-scan, we will be able to move on to hormone therapy and no more chemo EVER.

Yvonne, a lady at my church had a recurrence and had to do more chemo starting last week. I hope I am being blessed and I won't need to do any more than the hormone therapy and will live another 40 years cancer free.

March 30, 2010: Cycle number three is today. Only one more to go. The oncologist wants me to stay home on Friday, in part, because I am so tired, but mostly because I have no immunity and they don't want me exposed to whatever germs or viruses are out there.

I arrived about the same time as two other women and four more arrived shortly after that. They all left long before I did. Their treatments were only half hour doses, where mine is one hour and one and a half hours. After I got home, I had to lay down for an hour and a half, although I didn't actually. The nurse practitioners said I should start taking my blood pressure on Thursday and, if it drops, sort of play it by ear as to whether or not to take my BP meds.

April 10, 2010: Three cycles down and one to go. I hope when they do the CT-Scan, everything comes back clear. Chemo is rough. Yesterday, I talked to Tara's stepdad. He told me that Linda was going to stay with Tara while she was doing her chemo. When Linda called her, Tara told her that her next door neighbor is a Registered Nurse and would take her to chemo and help out while Tara is suffering the side effects of the chemo.

I told Vaughn that mothers always want to make everything all better for their children, but they can't always do that. Vaughn had to agree.

I was thinking that it is strange how things work out. Doug was retired before I had my mastectomy and able to do the cooking and helped with things like the laundry. I think the fact that he feels he is helping makes him feel useful since he can't fix my cancer. He keeps trying to feed me when I have chemo and I don't have the heart to tell him I don't feel much like eating the week after chemo, so I eat anyway.

April 20, 2010: Who would think that a volcano in Iceland would have a direct effect on me? My oncologist is stranded in London…The Carson Cancer center called me about 5:30 p.m. Saturday to reschedule my appointment. They wanted to move it up to Monday at 8:15 for the lab and 9:15 to see the other oncologist and then do chemo. That would wipe me out both Thursday and Friday, so I asked if we could go with a day later instead.

Since my chemo takes about four hours, they decided if I go in for labs at 11:30 and see the oncologist at 12:30, I should be finished about 4:30. That will work. God willing, this is the fourth and final chemo. Then comes the hormone therapy and after my system has a bit of time to settle down, a CT-scan. Hopefully that will be good.

I will need to see my primary care physician in June. By then, my current doctor will have moved away. I think I will try to get in to see a nurse practitioner whom I have seen before and who is now at a different office. Sometimes you deal with a medical person that you just feel understands where you are coming from and asks all the right questions.

Before Yvonne started chemo again, she told me she had gotten a wig when she did chemo the first time and wore it one day. She said that when she got home, her scalp hurt so bad that she couldn't lay her head on a pillow. I told her when my scalp felt that way; it was just before my hair fell out. Once that happened, my scalp felt okay and the wig didn't bother me.

Yvonne was wearing her wig Sunday. She said she was feeling pretty rough. She also told me that she had just gotten her hair back and now she has lost it again.

Tara started her chemo Friday. She will be doing a lower dose every week for 12 weeks. I should send her a note so she knows that I am still thinking of her. She is just beginning and I am finishing. I hope she is able to breeze through the chemo with few nasty side effects.

May 8, 2010: It's Saturday. After breakfast at Hy-Vee, I did laundry, hung out what I could and planted my Astors and Snapdragons. Then I helped Doug plant his garden. In two days, it is CT-scan time.

A part of me wants to believe no more chemo, but you know that the other little devil on the other shoulder, the one that keeps saying "are you sure?"

It sounds like Arland will have three cycles of chemo, then one of radiation, followed by three more cycles of chemo for his cancer in his brain.

Tara has had three cycles of chemo and is doing okay. After I find out what is next for me, I will write to her again. She is starting to shed her hair on about the same schedule as I did.

May 9th will be the third anniversary of the end of treatments for my cousin Lavon's colon cancer. Unfortunately her brother, Charlie, is losing his battle with esophageal cancer. No more radiation, chemo or surgery for him. He was basically sent home to die.

I am hoping for the best, but I can't quite be entirely positive. I am realistic enough to know that not all women with breast cancer breeze through treatment and that is the end of the cancer, except for hormone therapy. Of course, they only scheduled four cycles instead of six cycles like most of the women have had that I have talked to have had, so maybe I will be lucky. Time will tell.

May 11, 2010: Yesterday, I had a CT-scan at 8:30 a.m., then met with the oncologist at 11:15.

The 9mm spot on my liver was still 9mm. That is what they wanted. If it had grown or shrunk, that would have indicated the possibility of cancer, but it stayed the same, so they think it is probably nothing to worry about. NO MORE CHEMO!!! That is the best news I could have.

They put me on Femara, since the tumor tested 2% positive for the protein for hormone positive early breast cancer. I have to see the oncologist in a month and then every three months, with another CT-scan in six months. They will monitor the liver for two years and if the spot doesn't change that will confirm it is harmless.

I need a Dexa-scan to check my bone density, since Femara can cause bones to thin. They will schedule Dexa-scans every 2 years to monitor the effect the hormone therapy will have on my bones.

May 12, 2010: Arland started his chemo yesterday. He seemed to do okay according to Nancy. She wanted to know what to expect. I told her time would tell how he would react and some of the symptoms, that if they happen, not to worry.

May 12, 2010: I am still smiling, I think my oncologist fully expects that I will have no problems and will live to a ripe old age, but they do need to keep checking. I wouldn't have it any other way.

May 17, 2010: Tomorrow will be four weeks since my last chemo treatment. In other words, it is six days past what would have been a chemo day. I am starting to get my senses of taste and smell back. My feet and fingers are starting to feel better. I wonder how long it will be before I can actually see that my hair is growing back.

When I rub my head, I feel like there is a bit of re-growth starting. I hope the oncologist will agree to have the port removed. It is a pain. If I have to put up with it for a year, I won't be too happy about it, but I'll do it if I have to.

Arland wasn't happy about how the chemo wiped him out over the weekend and his port is still tender. My port incision is a neat little line and Arland is ragged and puckered. No wonder it hurts.

May 18, 2010: When I see the oncologist on June 7, I will ask about getting rid of the port. A year of maintaining it will be such a hassle.

May 24, 2010: I had my Dexa-scan today. Gail called this evening. She's having gall bladder surgery on the June 7th, the same day as I see my oncologist. I hope the Dexa-scan will show good bone density. If I don't have normal bone density, Gail will gloat because hers is great.

May 27, 2010: I went to my hairdresser today. It's been 37 days since the last chemo. The little bit of hair that I didn't shed has started to grow and is about one and a half inches long. The hair at the bottom of the back and over my ears seems to have the most re-growth. I sort of hated to have Lori buzz, since there is so little of it, but I think it will be easier if I don't have those few longer hairs sticking out of the rest.

May 31, 2010: My hair seems to be getting thicker all the time. It will be a while until I have enough to go out in public bareheaded. The wig is hot. The hat is hot. The scarves are a little better, but they are still hot.

June 9, 2010: Gail is doing better than I did after gall bladder surgery. She came to Norfolk today and two days after my gall bladder surgery, I left the bed and moved to the couch.

My oncologist said my bone density is a little bit sub-normal. I don't have to go back to the oncologist until September. I do need to get my port flushed in July and August.

I will need a Dexa-scan every two years, a mammogram annually, and CT-scans every six months for two years. I will be on hormone therapy for five years.

June 19, 2010: I keep rubbing my head to feel the new hair. I know that it will come back, but I'm impatient. Although there is quite a bit on the sides and back, it is only about ¼ inch long. The top is ¼ inch long but it is sparse. I am guessing by the time I am comfortable going bareheaded, it will be cold out. I will have to cover my head while it is hot. Well, I will just have to do what I need to do. If I have conquered the cancer, this is no big deal. My health is much more important than hair. I have a hat, two scarves, and a wig. They are hot, but I can make it through that.

I am starting to go bareheaded in the house and I took off my scarf while sitting under the tree in the backyard. I must admit I am starting to reach a point where I really don't care too much about how people will respond to a female baldy.

I was initially somewhat concerned that other people wouldn't be comfortable and I didn't want to cause that. Now I am comfortable with the hair loss and in a way almost proud of it. It is sort of like – to me it is a badge that says, "I am a cancer survivor."

June 25, 2010: Yesterday I was wandering around the neighbor's garage sale bareheaded. It was just too hot for even the scarf. I am getting a little more hair all the time. I wonder when I will be comfortable going out everywhere, bareheaded, no wig, no scarf.

June 26, 2010: I am getting more hair all the time. The sides, and back, although very short, have enough hair to cover the scalp. The top is a bit longer, but nowhere near as thick…All it wants to do is stand on end. That includes the short hairs on my arms and even my chin hairs are really soft.

July 2, 2010: My hair is getting thicker. The sides and back are nice and thick and the top is slowly filling in. I still have an area on top that is thin.

July 6, 2010: I have been going bareheaded in the house for a couple weeks and outside at home for a week. It was hot enough that when I got in my car at work, I just took off the wig and didn't put it back on when I got to my church women's group. It probably won't be too long before I start going bareheaded most, if not all, of the time, definitely before I see my oncologist in September.

July 10, 2010: Saturday – I went to breakfast this morning bareheaded. I am a little surprised at the lack of reaction I get from people. A few take a second look, but I guess there are enough chemo baldies around that they know what is going on.

Actually I am not completely bald. It is getting fairly thick except for a small area about the size of a deck of cards just above my forehead and that is getting smaller, closing in from all sides. It won't be long before I will have a good covering of hair. I have started to go bareheaded everywhere except to work. I will wear the wig there for at least a while.

My eyelashes had thinned some, but not too bad. Now that I am starting to get new growth, all the lashes that I hadn't lost, shed to make way for new lashes. I can't see them yet, or put mascara on them, but I can feel them. I do wonder what my hair will be like. It is all grey now and has a tendency to stand up and then curl, although it is still too short to know for sure.

July 11, 2010: Six months ago I had my mastectomy. It's almost the time of day that Gail left and I started one, long, miserable night. A lot has happened since then. I hope the next six months will be good.

July 20, 2010: My lashes are coming back thick. They are real short, but I have been able to get some mascara on them. My eyebrows are coming back and, unfortunately, my chin hairs are back, too. At this time they are soft, but I think I have twice as many as I used to.

Arland was given the choice of once a month chemo for a while, or taking his chances of having a recurrence. I think he is doing the chemo. He has a CT-scan this week and will have to see how it comes out.

September 10, 2010: Yesterday I had an appointment with my oncologist. On Tuesday, September 7th, I had lab work and they had a terrible time getting the backflow from the port. I guess there is a cancer marker that they can find in the blood for breast cancer. The test came back good. They wanted to schedule the CT-scan and mammogram to November, but had to settle for December 8th. If that comes back good, I will be able to get rid of the port. That will be great. So far, so good. I don't want to get overly optimistic because this is cancer, but with any luck I will be around to make it to 98, yet.

September 12, 2010: I was thinking that some women would be upset about having a mastectomy when it turns out that the tumor was under my right arm. I feel that it was the right decision for me. The day before my surgery, I was given a prayer shawl at church. Even though I had slept well the night before, I sat down to watch TV and since it being January, it was cool. I covered my body with the prayer shawl and fell asleep for about 45 minutes. When I woke up, I had two hot spots. One was the lump under my arm, That one was kind of a double (4cm tumor and 1.1 Lymph node) The other was a spot close to the breast bone where I had a cyst a number of years ago.

Both areas, besides being hot, were very tender. After a couple hours, I couldn't find the center one. I have a feeling that even though they didn't find anything there, that something would have developed later. Because under the arm is a very rare place for breast cancer to develop, the mammogram was basically normal. I was not a candidate for immediate reconstruction. Had I been I would have opted for a breast reduction on the left breast and an implant on the right side. Since we couldn't start reconstruction right away, I have chosen to not have any more surgery, which means I will live with Big Bertha and Phony Fiona for a long time.

October 8, 2010" I had my port flushed yesterday. My oncologist was there and wanted to know how I was doing on the Aromisin. In September, they switched me to Aromisin, since I was getting very achy on the Femara.

November 6, 2010: I finished the third pink prayer shawl today. I have been doing cards to go with them. The notes are handwritten and no two will be exactly alike. Some things are similar. I tell them that I, too, have heard the dreaded words, "You have breast cancer." I also tell them that I started making prayer shawls after I finished chemo and that I hope they do as well as I have. Maybe the fact that the shawl is from someone who has been through what they are facing, will somehow give them strength and comfort. I want to make a shawl for Arland next. He has lung cancer, which is another kind of cancer, but still it is cancer. I hope it will give Arland strength and comfort, too. I am pretty sure it will mean alot to Nancy.

This has been very hard on Nancy. I try to be there to listen to her and encourage her. She probably needs all the friends she can get who will be there to listen and care.

November 7, 2010: Dottie, from my church's Prayer Shawl Ministry, brought me some off white yarn for Arland's prayer shawl today. I started working on it this afternoon. It will be smaller than the ones I have been doing. If I work hard at it, maybe I can get it done by next weekend. I want to get it to Arland as soon as possible, rather than to wait four weeks. I'll have to check if it is okay to just give it to him or to first have it blessed.

November 21, 2010: I talked to my pastor and he said it is fine to take Arland his prayer shawl right away. It would still go with many prayers. I took it up on the 16th to Arland at the Doctor's Building. He surprised me by using words like "it's beautiful" and "it's gorgeous". I talked to Nancy Sunday night and told her that I had a prayer shawl for Arland and she told me when and where Arland would be for his chemo.

I stayed about 45 minutes. Arland thanked me a half a dozen times. Most telling of all was as he was talking to me; he was caressing the shawl and feeling the ripples. I think I received as much as I gave. At least I hope Arland gets as much comfort and peace as I did from mine.

I knew it would mean a lot to Nancy, but I was a bit surprised that Arland expressed so much appreciation. Most men don't. When I started making prayer shawls, I had hoped that someone would be really touched and be comforted with one of the shawls... Now I know that it has happened at least one time and could happen many times. Maybe not every time, but if it means as much to a few people as it did to me, then it is well worth it.

December 9, 2010: One year ago today, I went to my primary care doctor for a six month med check. I asked about a lump under my right arm. It turned out to be breast cancer. Today when I went to my oncologist, they said the CT-scan was great and the blood test for a cancer marker that signifies an active tumor growth was so good that they may not do CT-scans every six months for the two years.

I told them about my cat Baxter, beginning around August 2009, he started sticking his nose under my arm. He actually started doing that before I knew I had a lump there. In October or November, he started trying to bite the lump, getting more persistent as time passed. After I got home, following my mastectomy, he got on my lap and sniffed under my arm then left and wouldn't even sit on my lap for a week.

I told the P.A. that Baxter wasn't sniffing or biting anywhere, so I guess means I passed the CAT SCAN! Now the question was, did I pass the CT-scan? I did. So what did Baxter smell?

I don't have to go back to the oncologist until March and they scheduled an appointment with my surgeon for next Monday, December 13th, to get rid of the port. Yippy!!! They remove the port at the doctor's office with a local anesthetic. I was expecting to have to go to the surgical center like I did to have it put in.

December 23, 2010: On Monday, December 13th, I was De-ported, as my pastor said. After numbing it with Lidocaine, the surgeon took it out at his office. My flesh had attached itself to the port, so it would end up being tug, tug scrape, scrape, tug. Tug, scrape, scrape, etc. It probably sounded worse than it was since it was so close to my left ear. It did take about a half an hour and it was a bit more work than usual. I was bruised for 2 or 3 inches from the incision and needed more stitches than the surgeon said I would have, but by now most of the bruising is gone and most of the incision is healed.

The outside end of the incision is not quite healed and you can see the end of the subcutaneous stitch. It will dissolve and feels better every day. It has gotten to a point where it feels better than the port did. I wonder if the port was such a pain because of how it grew attached. Well, it is gone and I am happy.

Epilogue

September 2, 2012: Two days after I got rid of my port on December 13, 2010, my brother, Doug, went to the doctor because he was short of breath. After many tests, X-rays and a CT-scan on December 27, 2010, he was diagnosed with asbestos related lung cancer. Baxter had started avoiding Doug a few weeks before that for no apparent reason.

In May of 2011, Doug was briefly in remission. Baxter would sit on the end table next to him to be petted. By the first of June, Baxter would panic if Doug got anywhere near him. Not long after that, Doug's belly started to swell. On July 12, 2011, the VA hospital did a CT-scan. The cancer was back and it was angry. He died on July 27, 2011, exactly seven months after he was diagnosed.

Arland is still undergoing treatment, but is doing fairly well.

Yvonne lost her battle with cancer on June 30, 2012. She fought bravely for two and a half years, No matter how rough she felt, she always had a smile and did her best to take care of others. I will always remember her shining example of courage and how even when she was going through so much, she never felt sorry for herself.

Tara and I are both doing great. In June 2011, instead of a third CT-scan, I had an ultra sound of my liver. That was so good they extended the length of time between visits to four months.

On December 8th, when I had my mammogram, they found an enlarged lymph node under my left arm. On December 14th, they had me come back in for another mammogram and an ultra sound. After that I talked to my sister, Gail. She told me that if she used a liquid deodorant, her lymph nodes would swell up. So I got a solid deodorant. Three days after I started using it, I went in on December 20th for a biopsy of the lymph nodes, which were already shrinking. They did the biopsy anyway, just to be safe. The radiologist said that since several other family members reacted to the liquid version, it could very well be a genetic intolerance to a chemical in the deodorant.

Sisterhood of the Wounded Breast

My cousin, LaVon, also had a scare in December, but it turns out that her problems were because she is lactose intolerant and some of the meds she was taking contained lactose. My niece, Lynette, was tested for thyroid cancer in December and that came back clear. As a family we had three scares in December 2011, but we came back with the three out of three who were winners.

On December 23rd, at about 11:15 a.m., I got a call from the oncology office that the biopsy was benign and everything was completely normal, and to start packing for the cruise my oldest brother was taking his sisters on.

Chapter Fifteen

Beverly C.

My husband and I moved to Green Valley, Arizona from our longtime home in Nashville, Tennessee, in 2005. It was a big change to leave friends for a new home in the southwest.

In September, 2008, we celebrated our 50th wedding anniversary. My Maid-of-Honor came to celebrate the occasion so she was here to support me when I received a sudden diagnosis of breast cancer. During my regular annual physical, my doctor found a growth that felt slightly smaller than the size of my thumb's top joint. This lump showed up on my mammogram, but could not be seen on an ultra sound, so I was scheduled for MRI test. During the MRI a second lump was found beneath the first identified lump. When I saw the starburst spot on the mammogram, I knew it was cancer. That same week

Sisterhood of the Wounded Breast

I was diagnosed with shingles and glaucoma. Not a good week!

The next step was a needle biopsy. I received a call that the result was positive for malignancy and I was scheduled for surgery on September 27, 2008. The surgeon gave me treatment options, and I chose the option of a mastectomy on my left side. I had two sentinel nodes tested with the second coming back benign, while the first contained cancer cells. I was told, thankfully, that no cancer cells had breached the node wall. Because lymph nodes were removed, I do have lymphedema in my left arm. I have exercises to do for it and I have an elastic sleeve to wear. This keeps the swelling to a minimum. I decided against a double mastectomy and also any reconstruction. The morning following surgery, a nurse wanted to know what my pain level was on a grade of one to ten. She was amazed that I had no pain at all. I took one pain pill for the trip home from the hospital as a precaution, but it wasn't necessary.

I told my oncologist that I wanted to treat the cancer aggressively and he agreed that's just what we should do. He scheduled me for six chemotherapy treatments, two weeks apart, beginning the end of October. I was given stretching exercises to do with my left arm. Since the exercises were uncomfortable, I didn't do them regularly. Because I didn't do what I was supposed to, I wound up with a frozen shoulder and needed physical therapy to restore movement in that shoulder. My husband, and my daughter who lives in Tucson, went to every doctor appointment and every treatment and test with me. I would have my chemotherapy treatment and then go back for a shot on the following day to boost my white cell count. At first, during the week following a treatment, I had a couple days that I felt fairly well. But as the treatments progressed, that didn't last. I began to feel worse and experienced nausea, chills, joint pain and severe fatigue, to the point that I often had difficulty walking from the sofa to the bathroom. I was so fortunate that the timing of my "good days fell on Thanksgiving Day, Christmas Day, and during my Atlanta daughter's visit in January. Having since learned of many of the terrible side effects that sometimes follow chemotherapy, I feel thankful that I was spared so many of them.

After chemo, everything tasted like straw. I tried to eat a bit at every meal, but usually couldn't. My husband would go to Dairy Queen, Arby's or anywhere he thought might something that would taste good for me. My oncologist's nurse suggested I should eat a dill pickle before every meal. I tried it and it worked; some food then had some taste to it!

Another possible effect my audiologist said could happen, with the particular chemotherapy drug I was given, was a loss of hearing. However, I didn't notice that at all. The loss of my hair has been my most traumatic event. Two weeks, to the day, after my first treatment, on a Sunday morning, as I was getting ready for church, my hair came out in clumps. Thankfully, before my chemo sessions began, my Tucson daughter went with me to buy a wig. My daughter from Atlanta sent me several caps, one with spiky hair sticking out of the top, which I wear a lot.

After completing all my chemo sessions, I was given Arimidex to take for five years as a follow up treatment. Everything may have side effects, and I am told that about ten percent of those who take Arimidex never have their hair grow back. Unfortunately, I seem to be one of the ten percent. My dermatologist says my hair probably won't ever return, even after quitting Arimidex.

My husband was such a trooper and the best caregiver, ever. He stayed near me all the time, except when he had to go for groceries or other necessities. At the time, I didn't realize how hard all this was on him, too.

February, 2013, I reached my five-year anniversary of my diagnosis and last treatment. I was concerned about discontinuing my prescription of Arimidex. In my mind, those small pills were inside me working like little Pac-men, traveling around and eating any nasty cells. On what I thought would be my last visit with the oncologist, I was so relieved when he recommended five more years of Arimidex and would continue under his care. A recent study showed that ten years of Arimidex seems to improve the chances of non-recurrence in some women.

Though I would not want to go through the experience again, I am thankful that I had my yearly exams and the lump was not there on my mammogram the year before my diagnosis. I tell all my friends to do their self-exams every month and go for a yearly exam. I am emphatic and tell them to make it a priority.

Years ago, a friend, who was diagnosed with melanoma, told me that at first she thought "why me"? "I never smoked, I never drank and I lived a good life. But then I thought "why not me?" I know now how she felt.

The diagnosis of cancer changed my life. I feel I have since lost some of my self-confidence, and sometimes I still grieve over the loss of my hair. But I have always depended on my Lord and I felt His presence throughout this experience. I wake up every morning and say, "Thank you, Lord, for another day."

Chapter Sixteen

Carole S. Campbell, Ph.D.

Standing in the shower in my New Orleans apartment, I checked my breasts. Oh, oh. A small pea-sized lump caught my attention. I checked it, again, and again, but it WAS still there.

Quick calculations for my next trip to Seattle, I decided to make an appointment for a mammogram in less than three weeks. I kept feeling the lump and it didn't seem to change. As soon as I was home in Seattle, I had the mammogram. The news was encouraging, because although the technicians could feel it, the lump didn't show up on the mammogram. That, to me, was great news because, in my naivety, I thought that meant that I didn't have a problem with breast cancer. I was told to keep an eye on it and continue with my doctoral studies in New Orleans.

About six weeks later, I left New Orleans to drive back to Seattle alone. As I drove the almost 3000 miles in my little blue Toyota, I began to sense the breast wasn't quite behaving in its usual way. The first thing I noticed was that the right breast seemed a little reddish and a bit warmer than usual. There were also stabbing pains that I hadn't noticed earlier.

I arrived home mid-afternoon, six days later. Not wanting to alarm my husband, I waited until he went to get groceries, then I called my gynecologist. I could tell the office receptionist took me seriously, because they gave me an appointment first thing the next morning.

As the gynecologist checked, I could tell she didn't like what I was presenting. She tried to take a needle biopsy, but it was unsuccessful. She sent me to a surgeon for the biopsy and I waited for the results. About a week later, I heard about the biopsy and didn't like what I was told. I had breast cancer, Stage 3, Inflammatory.

Suddenly, I became the object of much interest by oncologists, who determined the treatment in advance and really gave me no choices. Because the tumor was so large, 9 cm. across, the oncologist didn't recommend surgery immediately. Instead, I was to have four "rounds" of chemotherapy. The purpose: to see how I and the tumor would react. At first, I didn't think I would lose my hair, but sometime after round #2, it started falling out. I sat in my back yard while the loose hair was brushed out, and the remainder clipped off. My hair has not grown back in the 18 years since that haircut. I think the treatment had to be very effective.

The four rounds of chemotherapy went by quite easily and soon I went "under the knife" for a mastectomy. Because my tumor shrank from 9.0 cm. to 0.2 cm across, I asked what I thought was a logical question – could I have a lumpectomy and be done? Their response was a resounding NO! In September, I had a modified radical mastectomy and became lopsided. I didn't like the arrangement, but it was workable and I lived with it for another 10 years. At least I didn't have to go through resizing the real breast to match the artificial one as a friend did, who chose to have a prosthesis implanted under her skin. I bought a "mastectomy bra", added the prostheses to one side and went happily along with my life almost as if nothing had happened. That condition was good for 10 years.

My left breast presented quite differently from the right. It became very tender and uncomfortable, but didn't seem to have any "lump". If it hadn't hurt, I probably would have passed on it, writing it off as something else. But, it wasn't. It was another way for a tumor to present itself.

This time was less intrusive because I reported the problem much earlier. However, the outcome was the same. I called myself fortunate because it was a "new primary", not a metastasis. That meant the original treatment was still in effect, but I probably have the BRCA-1 and BRCA-2 genes for breast cancer. It was clear that I should tell my brother, because he has two daughters who may also carry these genes. I did so, but I don't know if he did anything with the information.

Another mastectomy followed and now I used both pockets in the mastectomy bra. I was given a pair of breast prosthesis that was supposed to stick to my chest. I wore them for a while, but I found it a nuisance to wash them as meticulously as necessary, so I reverted to the originals, which don't require such tender, loving care.

Breast cancer is certainly no picnic, but like many things, it's manageable when properly treated. My biggest wish is that my special friend, Diane, would have had the option of the treatment I received and hadn't died of breast cancer at the age of 38.

Chapter Seventeen

Linda S.

During the time that I lived in Orange County, CA, I was a member of a Bible Study group for twenty years. This brought me to my first real awareness of breast cancer.

Our group leader, Gwen, had a mammogram, which was normal and clear, but four months later, she had a lumpectomy because of a very aggressive breast cancer diagnosis. Further complications caused her to undergo stem cell replacement, which involved thirty long days in isolation at the hospital. She recovered and was able to thrive for several more years, traveling abroad and working a full time job at her church, even though she developed a blood clot in her leg, deep vein thrombosis, thought to be a complication of her cancer treatment. Gwen was able to see her daughter get married and have the joy of her life – twin grandchildren – a boy and a girl. Shortly after their birth, Gwen fell victim to another complication from her therapy, leukemia, and she ultimately lost her life in 2005.

During Gwen's journey through breast cancer, our minister's wife was diagnosed with breast cancer and underwent surgery on January 11, 2002. She had a double mastectomy and reconstruction, and our church members helped her in every way that we possibly could. This included our prayer circle. Gwen, as our leader, asked each one of us if we were up to date on our mammograms. I was not – I was eighteen months out from my last mammogram. I basically had no health insurance, and was putting off a lot of routine medical procedures that would normally have been taken care of with insurance. With reluctance, I confided in Gwen and told her my situation. She did some research and gave me a phone number to call for a free mammogram. So, at Gwen's insistence, I called and set up an appointment. I received a callback for a second mammogram. It was in April of 2002, following a biopsy, when I received the diagnosis of cancer, DCIS in my lower left breast. I also had an ultrasound test which showed a second site of tubular lobular cancer up high in the left breast tissue. It was a star-like shape, with finger radiating out from the site. The discovery of two different cancers, and two separate sites identified, then mandated a mastectomy.

Sisterhood of the Wounded Breast

Earlier, I mentioned that "I basically had no health insurance." Actually I had purchased some supplemental insurance, but my coverage left me "very under insured". With only minimal health insurance coverage, who would have accepted me? That was the bad news. But, because of my under-insured status, my medical case was picked up by a Breast Cancer Treatment Program administrated by the state of California. The good news was, that this supplemental insurance that I had actually opened more doors to doctors and treatment.

The first surgeon looked at my previous mammogram taken eighteen months earlier and said my right breast looked just like the left one appeared at that time. He predicted problems in the future with the right side. He said with my being a big breasted woman, it was only a matter of time before a mastectomy may be needed on that side, too.

I was scheduled for a bilateral mastectomy in May, 2002. The surgery went fine, but two weeks later, I was back in the hospital with necrosis on the right side. I went back into surgery for removal of more tissue. I had expanders placed in the breast areas for reconstruction, but they didn't begin to fill them for expansion until the fall, during October and November. It was a very slow process.

Meanwhile, I attended a Breast Cancer Support group at the hospital and made some wonderful friends there. I met Marlene there, a very good friend with whom I still remain in contact. In January, 2003, I attended the regular group meeting. Some members attended regularly, but others came sporadically. At that meeting, one of the sporadic members told her story, saying that during her recovery, she had bright red spots appear on her skin. She had acquired a serious internal infection and those spots were a symptom. A couple days later, I noticed pink bruises on my chest and I called my doctor. I was told to go immediately for a blood draw and went back to the hospital for two days of high dose antibiotics administered through IVs. While at the hospital, a pic line was inserted in my upper arm and I was sent home with a portable pump to continue the infusion of antibiotics for two weeks. This was so serious that I was put under the care of a doctor who specialized in infectious diseases. I had to have multiple blood tests during that time to monitor the infection.

Back at the Breast Cancer Support group meeting, we all talked about how important it was that one member's story raised the awareness of symptoms for everyone. Participating in my support group may have saved my life.

In May, one year after the expanders were inserted, they were swapped out for permanent implants. The temporary tissue expanders had been placed high and in a long shape on the chest to stretch the skin, so that the permanent implants would hang correctly. Because I am a breast cancer survivor, I was able to have silicone implants for my reconstruction. Silicone implants are not legally allowed for cosmetic enhancement and saline implants are used instead. Because I am a big and tall lady, I had also been a woman with very large breasts. To accommodate my size, the largest round implants were used, but the rounded look was not right. Furthermore, because my right side had less skin as a result of the surgery for necrosis, the reconstructed breasts appeared very imbalanced with the left side looking much larger than the right side. So in August the surgeon did another revision to replace the round implants with smaller, tear-drop shaped implants, with the intention of placing the next smaller size on the left so as to balance the appearance of size. Unfortunately, that did not happen, and both sides received the same sized implants and the imbalance was perpetuated.

By now, my medical coverage under the Breast Cancer Treatment Program had expired and I no longer had medical insurance. During the previous 18 months of treatment, I was hospitalized five times for the four surgeries and had many visits to multiple surgeons; a plastic surgeon, an oncologist, other specialists, home health nurses, and several blood labs. I was so grateful for this coverage. The blessing was that my treatment included the original diagnosis of Stage 0 (zero) breast cancer, two mammograms, three needle biopsies, a double mastectomy, a revision to remove necrosis of the skin, treatment for serious internal infection, tissue expansion, and two reconstructive surgeries for implants. Because of my EARLY DIAGNOSIS, (stage 0), I did not have to undergo chemotherapy or radiation. But now that I was a "Cancer Survivor", the cost for new health insurance was prohibitive with a "pre-existing condition."

Again, I was without health insurance.

In 2009, I moved to Arizona and found a job with health benefits. I started having trouble with scar tissue which was constricting the silicone implants. This constriction made them hard and very uncomfortable. I had the implants surgically removed. This was quite fortunate and timely because the implant from the right breast was found to be leaking, with the leakage being totally contained within the scar tissue surrounding the implant. I chose to not have the implants replaced; instead I now take advantage of prosthetic breast pads.

I came to Green Valley, AZ, just south of Tucson, as I have a brother in Tucson, and now I have a sister, too, in Tucson. I wanted to be nearer my family. I had gone through a stressful divorce. When my Mom died a couple years before I was diagnosed with cancer, I handled her estate.

My motto became "A girl's gotta do what a girl's gotta do!" I just kept on doing.

I was thankful for the support groups, my sister, my wonderful friends and my church. I always knew the Lord was with me.

"Fear Not, says the Lord." And I believe that.

Chapter Eighteen

Suzy

In the spring of 1999, I became concerned that something was wrong with the nipple of my right breast, but we were so busy with our son's wedding and the arrival of my brothers from England, that I put it out of my mind. Following the wedding in August, I had my annual mammogram in early October and it came back negative. But I became increasingly concerned even though there was nothing visibly wrong. I finally scheduled an appointment with our family doctor who was also a family friend. He decided that, though there was nothing he could see, we should visit a surgeon whom he knew to find out what was going on.

He arranged an appointment for the following day and the surgeon decided to do a biopsy. The diagnosis returned as a diagnosis of inflammatory breast cancer at stage 2 or 3. I had never heard of inflammatory breast cancer and I was stunned. He explained what I had and what the process for my treatment would be. His positive attitude and willingness to give me all the time I needed, to ask questions, was invaluable.

When I asked him if I was going to die, he said, "Not if I can help it."

Due to the advanced stage of my cancer, he scheduled surgery for the second week of November with chemotherapy starting three weeks after surgery. I would have radiation following the chemotherapy. During the pre-surgery workup, they did all the tests to see if the cancer had spread to other areas of my body and, fortunately, they were all negative.

The surgery went well and there was no sign the tumor had spread. However, 13 of 23 lymph nodes were positive. Three weeks after surgery, we met the oncologist to whom the surgeon referred us. The oncologist explained that without chemotherapy, my odds were one in four for a five-year survival; with chemotherapy, they were three in four. This quickly changed my mind about the importance of losing my hair. He explained the process and the side-effects and suggested that we start immediately. When I asked him what I could do during chemotherapy, he replied, "You are not sick, the cancer has been removed and chemotherapy will kill anything floating around in your body. Do whatever you want to do."

And on that note, my journey as a breast cancer survivor began.

People have asked me many questions about why I chose the treatment I did. The answer is simple. I had a wonderful family doctor, who sent me to a wonderful surgeon, who sent me to a wonderful oncologist, who sent me to a wonderful radiologist. I did what they told me to do. Added to that, I had lots of love and support from my family and I chose to return to work within a month after surgery and kept my life as normal as possible.

So here I am in 2014, remembering the surgeon saying, "I know you won't believe this, but someday you will look back and this will all seem like a bump in the road."

Chapter Nineteen

Patricia A. Howard

I am from Kent, WA, where Relay for Life began in 1985. That was the year when Dr. Gordon Klatt ran and walked for twenty-four hours straight on a stadium track in Tacoma, WA. He alone raised $27,000 for the event. He became so weary and wanted to quit before the hours were up, but a doctor friend brought him chicken noodle soup to revive his determination and he continued to the end. His mantra for the twenty-four hour timeline was "Cancer Doesn't Sleep; Cancer Doesn't Stop," and he didn't either. His effort was to push the idea that "one man made a difference, now millions make a difference." And so was born the idea for the many annual Relays for Life with the survivor walk and luminaries in honor and memory of all those diagnosed with cancer.

Mary L. Maas

I started working with Relay for Life in 1990 before ever experiencing cancer myself. A friend was on the planning committee and asked me to help. So for the past twenty-three years, I have been acquainted with cancer.

We moved from Washington to Sahuarita, Arizona in 2005. I continued my involvement with the cancer fund drive of Relay for Life.

Because of those years of knowing and working with survivors, and hearing their stories, it really didn't surprise me when I was diagnosed with breast cancer, and I wasn't upset. I assured my family that I would be fine.

In 2011, around my birthday in mid-July, I was performing a self-examination when I found a lump on my right side, low on my breast in the bra line. I told my husband and he felt it and agreed that it was a lump. He said I needed to have it checked. On July 18th, I had an appointment with an oncologist in Green Valley, AZ. He checked my breast and sent me over to Rapid Sound for a mammogram. The assistant found the lump and tried to get it on the x-ray. I was to receive the results in a few days.

On the following Monday, August 1st, the doctor's assistant called and said the mammogram was normal. I asked to speak to the PA doctor about the lump and she ordered a breast MRI at Radiology, Limited in Tucson. One week later I had the MRI and was told I would get the results in a few days.

I received a follow-up phone call and was told the MRI indicated a lesion and I needed to have an ultrasound and biopsy. On August 22nd, I had the tests completed at Radiology Ltd. Once again I was told I would get the results in a couple days. I received the news two days later when my oncology doctor in Green Valley called me in the evening and said the biopsy showed cancer. I immediately called my minister and we prayed together over the phone. I didn't want everyone to know, but he said, "Prayer Works." He added my name to the Prayer Chain.

The doctor told me his office would make an appointment for a lumpectomy at Tucson Medical Center, TMC, and he recommended a doctor to do the surgery. I met with the surgeon on Friday, September 9th, and was told the lump was Stage 1 breast cancer. I was scheduled for an outpatient lumpectomy on September 20th at TMC. I had to have a bone density test, and EKG, and a chest x-ray before the surgery. I was to see my oncologist doctor three weeks after the procedure. I would begin radiation four weeks after the surgery to be given in daily treatments for six weeks from about October 18th through November 29th. Then I would have hormone therapy, or perhaps, but less likely, chemotherapy.

I had my lumpectomy on September 20th, 2011. It was scheduled for 8:30 a.m. and was to take about one and a half hours. The lump was encapsulated and the lymph nodes were clear.

My next step of my journey was to meet with the Radiation Oncologist at Arizona Oncology. He is in the same clinic with my oncologist doctor. The two doctors conferred and I was recommended for an ONCA test because of my possibility for future cancer. This test could not be sent to Medicare until two weeks following the surgery and the test results would take another two weeks. On October 21st, I met with my oncologist and the results of the ONCA test showed I was on the low end of the chart for recurrence. My oncologist recommended five years of a pill therapy which has proven to help stop the return of cancer. That afternoon I had a DEX scan, which showed a thinning of some of my bones.

Jack and I met with the radiation oncologist on October 24th. He drew out the progression of my breast cancer on the paper covering the patient examination table. He explained from the start of the cancer to the end of chemotherapy or radiation treatments and drew the diagram. He scheduled my first radiation treatment for October 31st. However, I had a touch of flu and ended up in an emergency room with pain in my left arm and back. I thought it had something to do with my heart, but the tests were negative, so I went home. I had shingles. Another doctor prescribed Famciclovir, but the pills made me ill. Then my radiation oncologist prescribed Gabapentin for the pain. The prescription worked and helped me sleep, plus it helped with my hot flashes.

I began radiation treatments on November 3rd. I finished with my last treatment on December 23rd 2011. I suffered no side effects from the radiation.

I met with my oncologist for a final visit on January 5, 2013. He still recommended that I take Femara tablet for five years despite the side effects of weight gain, joint aches and an increase in my cholesterol level. He told me to continue on the Gabapentin for control of hot flashes, which may continue indefinitely.

I had to schedule a mammogram, or preferably a breast MRI in 4–6 months following the end of radiation treatments. I would have to see the PA in oncology every four months for a while.

I believe the main thing to do is listen to your body. If you see or feel anything suspicious, have it checked out. Another thing is to not keep it to yourself. My husband was such a great support. He went to every appointment with me.

Chapter Twenty

Deb

At the time I found my lump, I was going through a lot of stress in a divorce. I had very dense breasts and in January, 2002, I was diagnosed with Stage t3n1, a very large tumor and compromised lymph nodes. My OB-GYN sent me to a surgeon who confirmed the diagnosis of cancer.

I needed to have a double mastectomy because of the large size of the tumor and the possibility of another tumor showing up. With the double mastectomy and reconstructive surgery, I decided I could have a matched pair of breasts and in the size I wanted. Following the initial surgery, I had to do six months of chemotherapy, but no radiation. I had my chemotherapy treatments scheduled for Fridays and could recuperate over the weekend. For the first two weeks after the chemotherapy, I developed flu-like symptoms. Then through the third week. I felt good and I could eat well, before undergoing another chemotherapy treatment. I went through a bad year and a half of these treatments.

I also had to deal with the loss of my hair after the first 4-5 days. I thought, okay, I can be a victim of this disease, or I could take a positive attitude. I chose to get my head buzzed and went and got a really cute wig. I decided my hair would grow back, which it did, and it came in quite kinky. I started to take daily walks and decided to take charge of my diet and eat healthier. I was going to take care of me.

I was given a prescription for Tamoxifen, which caused an unwelcome fifteen pound weight gain. After three years, I was given a new prescription for Femara, an aromatase inhibitor, for five years. The extra fifteen pounds disappeared with the change in medication.

I did find that the reconstructive surgery was much worse than the original mastectomy surgery. I had to deal with the tubes and dressings which had to be changed daily. I left the hospital and three days later, I contracted a horrible infection identified as Clostridium-difficile, commonly called C-diff. I also suffered from severe back spasms and had to use pain killers and muscle relaxants to help alleviate the pain. I took Vicodin which simply masked the pain and didn't help to find the solution for my problems.

I was a first grade teacher in Washington State when I went through the surgeries and the treatments. My students didn't seem to take any note of my wig or any changes in me.

When I first met my new husband, I told him right away about my experience and my new bosom. I was determined not to be a victim to cancer. I am a strong person and I know people get well after cancer. I do have some residual "chemo brain" issues and my memory is shot, but I refuse to think in the negative. I want to remind everyone to think positive thoughts and you will be okay.

Chapter Twenty-One

Rita Robinson Brown

Although I was 63 and I'd had my annual gynecologist's examinations and mammograms since my early twenties, I'd never been diagnosed with cancer. The post card reporting the results of my last x-rays noted a possible problem in my left breast and suggested further examination. I was irritated when I had to return to The Cancer Center for a second series of mammograms. Naked to the waist, I braced myself before the humongous metal machine and surrendered my breast for what seemed like torture. Even though I wasn't disciplined spiritually, I began to pray for the x-ray to reveal no problem.

As I waited for The Technician to return with The Radiologist's reading of the x-ray, I considered reasons why I couldn't have cancer. The Technician returned with The Radiologist's request for an ultra sound. Lying on the table, in a dimly lit room, I was witness to the procedure on a monitor.

Within the flickering black and white image, The Technician pointed out a dark spot, a tiny worm-like growth burrowing into my body. A biopsy was required to determine if I had a malignant tumor: the dreaded "C".

Within days, I met the first member of what would be "My Team", a group of specialist physicians, to treat my cancer: if indeed I had cancer. Dressed in civvies, like a cowboy, The Surgeon seemed far too casual to be serious about my having a deadly disease. After staring at my x-rays and manipulating my left breast, he dismissed me. I would have to return to The Cancer Center to have my needle biopsy. I was frustrated; I'd assumed he'd perform the procedure in his office and give me an answer on the spot.

Two days later, I returned to The Center. I'd been told I wouldn't need a driver after the procedure. Sure I was the victim of some HMO scam to require a series of expensive, unnecessary exams, I didn't trouble my husband with what I was up to. In another dark room for over an hour, I was poked with needles to render me "painless." I was blindfolded to keep me from watching Doctor Number Two, who said I'd hear six or seven clacking sounds like a giant stapler. When he zeroed in on "the spot", he said, "I'll leave a piece of metal, so we'll know where we're working." I wondered if the staples had been removed, but before I could ask he disappeared. The nurse had me crawl into a wheelchair to whiz down the hallway for another mammogram. I felt woozy as I stood before the open jaws of the mammo machine, and noted a bloody streak on the glass as The Technician arranged my breast before she "compressed".

The Technician at The Center assured me I'd learn the results of my tests by the end of the day, or in the morning at the latest. I hadn't the energy to ask if indeed I'd receive a call on Saturday morning. For this was Friday – that afternoon, I tried to snooze as I waited for the phone call, which never came. Then Saturday and Sunday dragged on with no contact. By Monday afternoon, I phoned Dr. N's office. No results had been returned. By Tuesday morning, I decided that I must be cancer free; no news was good news. As I whisked out the door for my Yoga class, the phone rang. Dr. N told me, "You have a tumor." I babbled about the good news. His voice was stern, "You have a malignant tumor; you have cancer." He ordered me to come into the office to see him and connected me with the receptionist. Before I could tell her that this was an error, she booked my appointment for the following day. Reading my panic, my dogs stared at me with compassionate, doggy brown eyes.

As I sped to my class, I prayed to the God of my understanding – a being I call my Higher Power – or in emergencies like this one, my H.P. "H.P.," I pleaded, "I can't have cancer." I rushed into the studio and my instructor asked, "How are you?"

I looked at her as if she could dissuade me of my news. "I have cancer," I said, and I began to cry.

What Happened

Because I'm an educated, well-insured woman, I decided to trust in western medicine. The Surgeon had suggested the possibility for three treatments, for which he could provide the surgical component: a mastectomy with a breast reconstruction at the time of the surgery and no radiation or chemotherapy required. The second option was a lumpectomy with an examination of the lymph nodes using a sentinel node. He defined the sentinel node technique as a new one, when one node is cast with dye and it's sent through the system to determine if others are affected. And my final Option, a lumpectomy, sentinel node check, chemotherapy and radiation.

My husband and I met with my third doctor, The Oncologist. We listened carefully to his suggestions. I selected what he termed the "aggressive panel." For my cure I'd have surgery with Dr. N. – the lumpectomy and the sentinel node procedure. Then I would have a series of four or five chemotherapy treatments, spaced three weeks apart over a four month period. This would be followed by radiation, probably thirty-five treatments on a daily basis for a month or so. Of course, all treatment would be altered according to the results of the lymph node involvement. The Physician's Assistant handed me a folder packed with informative brochures and phone numbers of support groups. One of the first slogans to register with me was "The best protection is early detection." I'd be labeled as a stage one and a half out of the possible four stages.

A reader and a student for most of my life, I read nonstop. Among my choices were Dr. Love's *The Breast* and Lance Armstrong's and Gilda Radnor's memoirs about their cancers. I also read the magazines distributed by The Cancer Center. I was referred to a psychologist, who was a specialist in treating chronic diseases. The woman is a stage IV breast cancer survivor. I saw her on a weekly basis during the years of my treatment and read her book about recovery. My husband and I visited Sunstone, a recovery center for cancer sufferers and their families. The Nutritionist suggested the cancer diet. So the Nutritionist at my health club designed my food plan, one I still adhere to today.

My surgeon determined that I had no lymph node involvement, so I began chemo. I practiced prayer and meditation as I sat in the chair for hours while the needle dripped the powerful cocktail of chemo and steroids into my body. My mantra was, "Breathe in God, Breath out fear."

A month and a half into my treatments, my hair began to fall out. My husband took me to a beauty shop, where my head was shaved. I didn't want to wear wigs, so I bought a bunch of scarves. The American Cancer Society held a cancer survivors workshop on makeup and wig styling. Volunteer Aestheticians assisted the cancer sufferers in applying makeup and we were given cosmetics and grooming tips. The Center connected me with a woman, who is an RN, who'd recently been treated for breast cancer. I phoned her for information and support about each of the phases of my treatment. She encouraged me not to surrender to the disease and explained how her connection to her spiritual beliefs had become stronger through her treatment. This also became true for me. I prayed and meditated daily, and I napped. After one particularly rigorous chemo treatment, I slept nonstop for twenty-two hours. My Oncologist said that was part of the therapy. My husband prepared meals for us, brought me tea and drove me to my appointments. And he always encouraged me to recover.

Near the end of my chemo treatments, I began to feel a bit energetic because of the steroids, anti-nausea drugs and shots for my anemia (those injections cost over three thousand dollars each) I joined Boot Cancer Camp for Breast Cancer Survivors. Weekly, I met with our Sergeant and a dozen or so women to exercise. We were given exercises to perform during the week and we kept a journal of our daily workouts. I was the Boot Camp graduation speaker, for I'd been the most committed to practicing and keeping a journal. My cancer free friends and my husband cheered after I gave my address.

After finishing chemo, I started radiation. I made a group of friends whom I saw everyday; some were technicians, some were fellow patients. By the end of my thirty-five treatments, I had developed the condition of folliculitus, and infection in the hair follicles. The itching stopped after I applied prescribed creams and ceased my radiation. The hair on my head began to grow back in soft, salt-and-pepper curls, fine as duck down. Friends asked permission to pat my hair. My beautician advised me not to put peroxide on my hair, "The jury's still out on the relationship to cancer."

I began the regime of medications, which were estrogen blockers.

What It's Like Today

I have celebrated nine years of remission. This state has required actions and effort on my part, and the unconditional support of "my Team", my husband, friends and my Higher Power. I have rigorously followed my physician's advice. The fourth doctor on My Team, The Radiologist, a petite young woman, suggested maintaining my ideal weight. The tumor which I had was estrogen sensitive and body fat in women creates estrogen. In addition to keeping within five pounds of my ideal weight for these past nine years, I completed the five years of medication to block the creation of estrogen. Two years after completing my cancer therapy, my Gynecologist suggested I have a hysterectomy and an offerectomy. The uterus and ovaries are often sites for cancer, and my uterus was filled with fibroids. I scheduled regular mammograms and appointments with my Oncologist to have blood work and examinations and to determine that I was cancer free.

To make a financial contribution for cancer research, each year I have attended the Susan B. Komen Race for the Cure. Surrounded by "Warriors in Pink," I celebrate my recovery and that of my fellow cancer survivors and pay tribute to those who've died of the disease. My brother-in-law was one of the one percent of men who suffered from breast cancer.

I have been ever vigilant for signs of cancer. The scar tissue from my lumpectomy was so thick; it was difficult to tell if another tumor was beneath the layers of skin. I had a second lumpectomy to clean up the scar tissue. Three years I developed a swelling in the incision where my lumpectomy was performed. The Physician's Assistant for my Oncologist explained that I had a Seroma; the pocket where my cancer had been and was now filled with harmless fluid. On three occasions, my P.A. removed the fluid and each time sent a sample of it for a biopsy. No signs of cancer were present.

The following year when I had my mammogram, the attending Radiologist told me having the Seroma drained was a greater risk than just leaving it alone. The Seroma has become smaller in the ensuing years. In addition to having my breasts x-rayed, I have had pictures of my lungs taken, too. If cancer doesn't return to the breasts, another site could be the lungs or any soft tissue.

Some of the side effects of cancer therapy have not been pleasant. I have had cataract surgery in both eyes. According to my Ophthalmologist, the cancer blocking drugs which I took hastened the development of cataracts. Because of the eye surgery, my eyes are dry and I must take expensive drugs three times a day to maintain their moisture level. The estrogen blockers have taken a toll on my skin. I am very fair and so thin-skinned that I bruise at the slightest touch and my skin tears very easily. I've experienced some bone loss but the drug to strengthen the bones was one that I had adverse responses to, so I rely on calcium supplements and exercise. I also take Turmeric and other supplements to strengthen my immune system. My breasts are not symmetrical and differ about two cups sizes from one another. My scar is deep so the nipple is aimed to the side, not straight ahead. I could have elected to have reconstructive surgery, but I chose not to. One of my best friends is a professional bra fitter who helps me purchase a variety of prosthesis and a number of beautiful bras. My Oncologist writes an annual prescription for these carefully designed pads and attractive garments so Medicare pays a portion of the cost.

Every day when I wake, I am grateful for modern medicine and its practitioners, my insurance plan, and my troops of supportive friends, all of which have helped me and have helped in giving me a second chance to live. I am most grateful for the lessons cancer has taught me; Life is fragile and precious, and one must often rely on powers greater than oneself.

Chapter Twenty-Two

Janice/AKA: Oz

The year is 1994, married to Gene Oswald, a hard working farmer and I am a mother of four beautiful children who have become my whole world. Ryan is 16, Jennifer is 14, Kandace is 10 and Jacqueline is 7.

Hello! My name is Janice Oswald and I was born in Albuquerque, New Mexico on September 30, 1958. I was adopted by my wonderful parents, Marvin and Leota Heller, who are originally from Pilger, Nebraska. I was adopted when I was three days old and the minister from our Presbyterian church was the person who brought me home. Back in those days, when you adopted a baby, you went to the hospital, and you were allowed to look at all the babies who were placed for adoption, and you picked out the one you wanted. How special is that!

Mary L. Maas

When my parents told me the story, when I was old enough to understand, it made me feel so Special and even more loved. They have always been the most amazing parents anyone could ever ask for. God must have known from the very start that I would really need them through this journey. I love you both, Mom and Dad.

I also have one brother, Michael Heller and he, too, was adopted at five days old. He is also very special to me and has been there whenever I asked. I love you, too, Mike. We lived in Albuquerque until I was halfway through the 6th grade, then we moved back to my parents' home town of Pilger, NE, where they purchased the Heller's I.G.A. Grocery Store.

Now back to 1994: Everyone was in school and we were busy running to some sort of school or sports event much of the time. Towards the end of August, I had fallen down a flight of stairs in our house. I'd heard Kandace screaming just after I thought they had all loaded on the bus for school. I was trying to hurry rounding the top of the staircase and I lost my balance and fell. I got up and hobbled outside to find Ryan chasing the dog who had taken off with Kandy's shoe.

In addition to bruises and bumps, I found out I had a torn rotator cuff on my right shoulder. I had rotator cuff surgery with many physical therapy sessions.

Sisterhood of the Wounded Breast

One day while taking a shower, I felt a pea-sized lump on the right side of my right breast. I was washing under my arm very carefully due to the surgery, and I thought, Hmm, what in the world is that. Could it be scar tissue? I'd never noticed it before, and I didn't think too much about it, and actually I kind of blew it off. I kept noticing it during my showers and thought it was becoming more noticeable, but I thought it had to have something to do with my surgery. The lump was rather hard and seemed to move around whenever I touched it. The more I messed with it, it began to be painful. Once you find something like that, it seems to always be on your mind. I would go into the bathroom often to check out this foreign object that was growing in my body and I wanted to see if it was getting bigger or going away.

It was not going away. It was really scaring me.

November 28, 1994: I got up, had my coffee, and took a shower to go to physical therapy. The lump grew from pea-sized to walnut-sized in a matter of about two weeks time. Then it hit me: Why would it be scar tissue on the side of my breast when the surgical site was on top of my right shoulder? Now I was really scared. I got dressed and headed to Norfolk. I asked the physical therapist what she would suggest and she agreed with me that I should call my doctor. I called Omaha and they could see me the next day to do a mammogram. I'd had my first mammogram in October of 1993, so they would be able to compare the two exams.

I called my best friend, LaRene, who is my sister-in-law, and asked her to ride with me. We had so many doctor bills at that moment and I didn't want Gene to know that I could possibly have another health problem, or that it may cost a bunch more money. We drove to Omaha and the doctor checked me over and sent me for another mammogram. The machines were not working so we had to reschedule for November 30. We returned home and I decided to tell Gene I had found a lump and had to go back to Omaha for a mammogram. He was very concerned and was glad I was going for an appointment.

Morning arrived and brought another surprise. Two of my best friends, Val and LaRene, were able to go along and whose support I really needed. We headed for Omaha and had the mammogram. We were told the radiologists would be able to read the mammogram right away and that we could wait.

It seemed like forever, but finally a nurse took me into a suite to wait for a doctor. Dr. H came in and told me he was very concerned and that I had a very suspicious lump which had been confirmed by the radiologists. He did not know if the lump was benign or malignant. I was crying and had no idea what he was telling me. He told me not to worry and he was sending me to a specialist. He was very caring and kind. He tried to make me feel better but it didn't seem to help.

I was a nervous wreck... My thoughts were racing. I couldn't move. My legs were like Jello. Do I have cancer? Am I going to die? Oh, my God, what am I going to do? The room was getting smaller and smaller. I wanted my Mama and she had no clue that I was in Omaha for this reason. She was taking care of my kids and was unaware that I had found a lump. Oh, boy, I knew I had to get myself together in order to even walk out of that room before I lost it. I made it to the waiting room, where LaRene and Val were waiting for me. They could tell by the look on my face that things were not okay. I tried to explain what the doctor had told me but I started to cry and I couldn't say the words. I was his last patient for the day and we were the only ones left in the office. Thankfully, Dr. H. noticed how upset I was and came over to explain the seriousness of the situation. He had scheduled me for the next morning with Dr. S. R. for a biopsy procedure.

December 1: We girls decided we would get a hotel and stay the night in Omaha, since we had to be here for my appointment the next morning. I was so thankful to have my two dearest friends with me. Getting a hotel room then became an adventure in itself. The front desk manager said there was only one room available. We took it. We walked into the most disgusting, filthy, unfit room imaginable. Val decided to return to the front desk to talk about getting a different room or we were leaving for another hotel. While she was gone, we made phone calls home, made arrangements for our families and talked to our kids. When Val returned to the room, we couldn't believe they'd somehow found another room for us. Val had already gone and checked it out and it was perfect. Imagine that.

Our next adventure was to go out to shop for p.j.s and to buy another set of clothes, etc. So off we went shopping and to have a bite to eat. I didn't eat much as I was nervous about having the biopsy the next morning. I couldn't believe it was the beginning of December and instead of looking forward to Christmas shopping, I was staring at rounds of doctor appointments and who knew what else.

I spent a very restless night. I had been instructed not to eat or drink anything after midnight, so I drank plenty before that time. The next morning, we headed to meet Dr. R. After we arrived, the nurse called me back and asked a few questions, took my vitals, and said Dr. R. would be in. He was really a nice man, very kind, and answered all my questions without making me feel uncomfortable in asking them. He said, "no question is a dumb question". After looking at my mammogram and examining me, Dr. R. informed me that we definitely needed to do the biopsy. He left the room and the nurse returned with this Little Paper Gown and asked me

Sisterhood of the Wounded Breast

to change into it. Now, first of all, I was thinking - where is the rest of it? Really! Oh, my! Excuse Me – Do you have these in a larger size? But I put it on and got back on the table, feeling like a whale in a Barbie dress! I was more than embarrassed when Dr. R. and the nurse returned. The nurse could tell and she was so nice, she asked me if I just loved the new designer gowns they'd just gotten in. Then she said not to think anything of it as it would not take long and she would be with me the whole time.

The needle Dr. R. brought in was about 12 inches long. He showed it to me and said they would numb the area and then with each piece they take out, it would make a loud noise and may hurt a little. The biopsy machine looked like a funnel with a needle attached. Well of course it was going to hurt. A needle of any length is going to hurt, never mind a twelve-inch needle. The nurse held my hand and talked continuously to help me remain calm. LOL—not working! I felt blood running down my side. He took five samples and then stitched and bandaged the biopsied area. They gave me an ice pack and told me to keep it on the area to help lessen the pain I would feel once the numbness wore off. After the procedure was finished, they helped me sit upright and the nurse asked me how I felt. I told her I felt dizzy and wondered if it because I hadn't eaten much since the night before. She said it could be that or the procedure itself. She gave me lemonade and crackers to see if that would help. I asked her to go get LaRene and Val to be with me. When they walked in, LaRene said I looked as white as a ghost.

Dr. R. came back and said they should have the results by the next day. We girls had to make a decision whether to spend another night in Omaha, or go home and return the next morning. We decided to go home and return as we all wanted to see our families. We stopped for a bite to eat and by then the numbness had worn off. The ice pack was no longer cold and the pain in my breast was throbbing. Our waitress was so kind and filled a zip lock bag with ice for me to use on the trip home. Great…tomorrow I find out if I have Cancer or Not. That was the only thing going through my mind. That Word Makes Me Sick.

December 2: That night I got very little sleep due to my constant worrying. Everyone kept saying I shouldn't worry and tried to reassure me that it was most likely nothing. They also said my odds were great because I had discovered the lump early. Dan and LaRene, Gene's brother and his wife, drove Gene and me back down to Omaha to be with us for moral support. It seemed like the longest trip to Omaha I had ever made. My appointment was at 1:50 and we were called right to the back. I got to change into one of those Cute, Little,- yes, LITTLE Paper designer gowns that they provide you with and let me tell you, there is nothing left to the imagination. Dr. R. came in and the first thing he said was "are we still friends?" I said "Of course, but I still hate the designer gowns." We laughed together.

I introduced him to Gene. Dr. R. told me he was sorry for any pain that may have occurred during the biopsy. He sat down on his stool, faced me and said, "You know, you are so young and generally people your age don't have to receive this kind of news. I regret having to tell you, your biopsy shows you have breast cancer." I remember his saying he was really sorry and he was talking, but My Whole World Fell Apart and tears were rolling and rolling and rolling! I couldn't believe it!

Oh My God, I have cancer. I hate you cancer. Everyone had convinced me that it couldn't be. I started sweating and shaking. My mouth was quivering uncontrollably and my nose was running. Gene seemed extremely upset and I knew he had no idea what he should do. I couldn't focus. Dr. R. felt so bad and handed me some Kleenex. All three of us had tears falling. That is how special Dr. R. is. Finally Gene had to ask the questions and Dr. R. explained everything in detail to us. I didn't even know what benign or malignant meant, or what mastectomy or lumpectomy meant. Chemotherapy? Radiation? Dr. R. drew diagrams on a paper for us which really helped. Time stood still that day and the hour that we were in there seemed like eight hours. Once Dr. R. explained in depth our options, we chose the route we both agreed would be the best. Surgery was set for December 7 at the Methodist Hospital in Omaha, for a right breast lumpectomy with removal of lymph nodes.

Gene and I returned to the waiting room where Dan and LaRene were waiting. We sat down and told them the bad news and we explained the details of the route we were going to take. We all were sick and couldn't be more afraid. My surgery was days away. We walked two blocks across the parking lot to where the hospital was located and started my pre-op tests. The initial paperwork was difficult to fill out as more and more of the questions didn't seem to pertain to me. The nurse came in to find me crying and she offered to help me. I told her I was unable to answer the questions, as I was adopted when I was three days old and I didn't know my medical history. She took the forms and said it was not a problem. She was an amazing R.N. and I wish I remembered her name as she was the best ever. What a dumb question, she remarked, #1. Do you live in a house…Hmmm…No. She lives in a tent on the ground…Duh. She had us laughing all the way through the questionnaire. Once we had finally completed my pre-op, I was told I could go home.

I couldn't wait to see my kids, but I wasn't sure how I would be able to explain to them that I had cancer. That was one of the hardest parts ever. Plus, all I was thinking about is whether the cancer may have already spread. Dear God, please let this all be a dream and wake me up. We went downstairs in the hospital to the lobby to call my mom and dad. That was another hard moment. They cried and assured me they would be there to help with anything I needed. I already knew that as they are the best. I was so glad that Dan and LaRene were with us as we couldn't have done it without their love and support.

December 3: This morning I told the kids. Ryan and Jenny looked so sad that it broke my heart. We all had tears and they looked like I had just ruined their lives. Kandy asked if I would lose my hair and asked if I was afraid. I told her I didn't know if I would lose my hair and I admitted I was kind of afraid. She said not to worry as I already had a green hat to wear and nobody would even know. She is such a character and I am so glad that she is. At that time I really needed that. It broke the silence and we all laughed a little. Then Jackie said, "I hope you don't die Mommy". She was only seven and we all cried again. This was too much for them and after telling them the bad news, I was exhausted. I took a shower and just stood under the spray and relived all the moments from the last few days.

What in the world just happened? I went from having a normal routine of school, games, church, etc. to a life of CRAZY. I was so angry that I didn't know how to handle this. What am I going to do? Lord, why is this happening? Did I do something to cause this? Where did the tumor come from? Could I have prevented this? What if it's all over my body? I never smoked or did drugs. I just stood there and bawled until the water grew cold.

Just a couple years earlier, Connie, one of the babysitters for the kids, was diagnosed with cancer while she was still in high school. The cancer affected her leg. She became very sick and lost her hair. We were all devastated as it was so hard to see her go through the treatments and such extreme ups and downs. She was like one of the family and we were so afraid for her. But she is a survivor today.

I remembered my first cousin Randy, who was also adopted. He was diagnosed with a malignant brain tumor at age 29. He had surgery immediately but they could not remove all of it. In time it spaghettied through his brain and he went through extensive treatments which caused psychotic episodes. He was seeing and hearing things which weren't real. He had to be placed in a mental care facility and then to a nursing home. At the age of 35, he was chosen King with his 85 year old Queen one Valentine's Day. He was confined to a wheelchair and later lost his battle at that young age of 35.

After close friends and family having experienced cancer, my diagnosis was scary. I prayed, Dear God, Please help me and help me through this. I can beat this. Amen. I repeated this prayer over and over.

In the next few days I visited several close friends to tell them of the situation. Kim and Deb were able to help me remain positive. A good support system and prayers became the most important things.

December 5: Val came over to help me call Dr. R. with a list of questions I had. She is an LPN and I hoped she could help me understand his answers. I wanted know if I had to have all the lymph nodes removed. When did I have to have the bone scan? If it spread, would I have the mastectomy right away after the lumpectomy? Did they do reconstructive surgery immediately? MRIs? And many more questions. I told him I had been researched everything I could find on breast cancer and how confusing it was. Dr. R. was so patient, answering all the questions and he calmed me down.

Everyone was concerned and our phone never stopped ringing. Talking to everyone was awesome, but it also gave me such anxiety. I cried often and I wanted to go to bed early so when I slept I didn't have to think about anything. One day, my friend Cindy called and I believe God must have sent her to call me. She helped me understand that I needed to snap out of my thinking about all the horrible possibilities and concentrate on the present. She said I had a tumor and it is called cancer. They would do surgery to remove that foreign thing. What we needed to do is to pray together right now. Over the phone Cindy prayed, "Dear Lord, please guide the doctors to do the very best they can do during the surgery on our friend, Janice. We also pray that the cancer has been contained, and has not spread into any lymph nodes, or to any other parts of her body. Please help Janice and her family to get through all of this, Lord, with your help. Help them to know you are there with them and to wrap your loving arms around them. We ask this in Jesus' name. Amen." Then she told me to let God know how I feel and to ask for his help. He will always be there for you whenever you need him, all you have to do is ask. I told her how afraid I was and that I wouldn't get to see my children grow up. She read some Bible verses to me and suggested I choose one thing each day; whether a person or a moment, that was special or bad, then pray about it each night. She said that was what she does and it makes a big difference in her life. So I took her advice and prayed for my family, for friends, especially for Cindy, that night.

December 6: It was snowing and we decided to head for Omaha early so we didn't get stranded. It was a good thing we did because the roads were not very good for our entire trip. Gene and I checked into our hotel room. While we waited for Dan and LaRene to arrive, we sat and talked and watched the snow fall outside our window. We realized the room heater wasn't working. We kept fiddling with the thermostat but the room remained cold. We called the front desk and they sent maintenance to check it

Sisterhood of the Wounded Breast

out. The heater was broken and we were moved to nicer room where the heater worked. When Dan and LaRene arrived they said the roads were horrible. We were glad they'd made it safely. That evening we went to the Red Lobster for supper and afterwards spent some time at the mall. We bought chocolates and coffee to take back to the hotel room. The snow was falling heavier and we were glad we came down early.

While everyone else slept, I was wide awake and my tummy was churning. I sat and watched the beautiful snow fall and prayed God would be with me and would guide Dr. R. to do his best. I slept about three hours before Gene woke me to get ready to go.

December 7: Surgery Day. The roads were crappy on the way to Methodist Hospital. I no more than checked in and was called back to be prepped for surgery. They wheeled me out to receive hugs and kisses from my family. LaRene held my hand and assured me everything would be okay. Gene told me not to be scared; he would be waiting for me. He gave me a kiss and told me he loved me and I went to surgery.

The surgical room was a little scary with the bright lights and huge silver, round-shaped equipment above me. Plus, it was really cold. Lots of machines had all kinds of buttons and lights, while IV bags hung ready and waiting. I wanted to run when I saw a table full of surgical knives and needles. Dr. R. came in and went over a few things with me and told me everything would be just fine. I told him I was scared but that I had complete faith in him and without realizing it, I was under. My surgery took about five hours with an additional hour in recovery. Gene was able to come and see me and told me Dr. R. was able to completely remove the tumor. The tumor was encapsulated and he was able to remove it before it spread. He said that it had fingers pressing against the sides, ready to push through. He removed all the lymph nodes from my arm and arm pit on the right side. He said it all looked good but they would send it in for further testing and we would find out the results in a couple days. Yea! Praise God and Thank you Dr. R.! I fell asleep while Gene was still talking and when I woke up I was in my room and my mom was by my side. I looked at her and the first thing I asked her was, "Do I still have my boob?" She said "Yes!" and we both burst out laughing. I had to look down my gown to make sure.

They gave me more pain medication which helped to keep me comfortable. Dr. R. came to see me the next day and had ordered a bone scan and more blood tests. He said everything looked good and that in a few days I was scheduled to see Dr. T. regarding my follow-up and to find out if I needed further treatment options. A few days later, I was released to go home. I still felt crappy, but couldn't have been more excited to see my kids and be in my own bed. They were all being so sweet to their mommy and I couldn't ask for better kids. I love them so much. They are definitely my world.

The week at home went by so quickly and before we knew it we were already heading back to Omaha. Gene and I arrived at the cancer center and checked in. The waiting room was packed full of people of many different ages and from all walks of life. We couldn't believe so many were affected by this horrible disease and while looking around the room, I noticed the large variety of wigs, hats and scarves used to hide hair loss. What scared me the most was seeing a few of them, who were as bald as a jay-bird and yet seemed 100% comfortable with not covering their heads. At that point I realized I had never felt so scared and have never been so nervous in my entire life.

The nurse finally called my name as it was my turn to be seen. While heading back, we walked through a room filled with people sitting in recliners, hooked up to all kinds of I.V.'s and monitors. I felt hot and dizzy. Walking further down the hall, I felt like I was going to pass out and had to grab Gene's arm and braced myself against the wall. They quickly got me into a room where I could sit down and gave me some water to sip. I began to feel better. I had never felt so overwhelmed. A few moments later Gene and I met Dr. T. Shortly after meeting him, he began to explain that he felt it was in my best interest to undergo chemotherapy and radiation, as a precautionary measure. One of the first questions I asked him was, "Will I lose my hair?" He told me as a result of the chemotherapy I would lose my hair and two weeks into my treatment, I would most likely be bald. Hearing those words made me sick.

Chemo was scheduled to begin in January of 1995.

December 29: A couple weeks shy of my first chemo treatment, we had a girl's day at Julie's, my sister-in-law. The girls and I discussed how I would soon lose my hair. Her sister, Steph, was there and mentioned how she thought it would probably be easier for me to deal with short hair falling out rather that a whole bunch of long hair. I agreed and since she is a beautician, I decided to take the plunge right then and there and let her cut off my long hair. There was a ton of hair falling to the floor and I had a hard time seeing it. I have had long hair for as long as I could remember. Everyone like the new cut and my husband joked with me and said, "Hey, I like your ears!"

January 5: Thursday morning, we headed down to Omaha to have a port surgically implanted into my chest, on the left side, leading into the main artery of my heart. It would provide easier access for an IV to administer the chemo each time. The surgery took a little over an hour and once I came out of recovery, they sent me up to the cancer floor for my first chemotherapy treatment. There I was introduced to all kinds of new medications and I didn't feel well at all. I was taking pain pills every two-three hours along with the IV nausea meds the given while introducing the new chemo drugs. That night I had to use nausea suppositories versus oral medications because I couldn't keep anything down. I was unable to eat the day I had my treatment as it made me nauseous. Even though the treatment made me very tired, the anxiety made it hard to get any decent sleep. I was very restless that first night and was up and down all night. This continued for the next couple days. I couldn't eat and everything smelled horrible to me. I smelled things that nobody else in the house could smell. I could smell the chocolate candy bars that were in their wrappers if they were anywhere near me and they made me feel ill. I remembered Connie, our babysitter, said that would happen to her, too, during her chemotherapy and no one else could smell those things either. I would ask the doctor about this. I was so tired and my anxiety was sending me over the edge.

January 7: Saturday - I was up and down and sick in the bathroom all night. I was a nervous wreck. I cried, I couldn't sleep; I couldn't eat and had hot and cold flashes. I called my doctor. I knew it was the weekend, but I couldn't wait. I was miserable and making everyone around me miserable, too. Dr. S. was the on-call physician for the weekend and he promptly returned my call. He had to listen to a woman who was out of control, sobbing and near ballistic, He was very kind and adjusted my meds I was on and added extra nausea medication. It didn't seem to help, I still was up and down all night long. My poor husband is such a gem for trying to help me cope with all this craziness.

January 8: The next morning I took some Compazine and waited a half an hour to take the Cytoxan, as Dr. S. asked me to and we went to church. Heaven knew I needed God right then and to get out of the house. Maybe going someplace where there were other people, I would think of something else. Church was good until the last 25 minutes and I suffered an anxiety attack, so we had to leave. We drove around so I could be outside and get some air, later we went to Gene's mother's home for a family dinner. Everyone from the Oswald family was there and that was so nice. There were 23 of us there and Gene's mom is a great cook. I managed to eat a little taste of roast, potatoes, corn and lettuce very slowly. When the dishes passed around the table, my anxiety returned and the bowls seemed like they were racing around the table as fast as they could go. By the afternoon, I was so nervous I went to lie in a guest bedroom, covered my head with a pillow and cried. Holding onto the pillow tightly was the only way things quit racing around me. Gene and LaRene decided we should call Dr. S. and hear his suggestions. By this time I had a severe headache and ear ache. Dr. S. gave me Xanax for the anxiety and Tylenol until I could be seen. Thoughtfully, the Wisner pharmacist opened up to get us the medication immediately and finally the Xanax helped me relax. I was able to get a good night's sleep as my friends were taking me wig shopping the following day. I needed to do this before I lost my hair. One of my friends had a sister-in-law who owns a beauty shop in Lincoln with a private room to try on wigs and buy them. I could have any color or style I wanted and tried on a number of them to model for my friends. It was like I was Marilyn Monroe until reality set in and I actually had to pick one out. I found one that looked like my own shoulder-length hair used to look. I put it on and had it combed and styled just like I used to wear my hair. Kim had left the room and when she came back she asked if I had found anything. We all began to laugh as she didn't even notice I was wearing a wig. It looked so real she'd forgotten I had cut my hair short. Perfect, I paid $49.84 and loved it. I had such awesome friends for support. Our day together was pretty good as long as I kept taking the Xanax and nausea pills. I was sick of the hot and cold flashes. The next day Dr. T. called to see how I was doing and prescribed Benadryl to my medications. He had spoken with Dr. S. and found out what a bad weekend I had. By this time I had lost around seven pounds due to my loss of taste for food. He said he would see me on the 12th for my next chemo treatment.

Val and LaRene went along to Omaha. I didn't want a needle poked into my chest as I still had the stitches from my port surgery. The area around my port was red and swollen so the lab had a nurse come down do the blood draw and to insert a catheter which she left in place for the chemo treatment.

During chemotherapy you sit in a recliner and they offer beverages, TV, and blankets. Your friends may sit with you. It took about an hour for the chemo to infuse. I had to use the restroom during the treatment and I saw the toilet was full of red liquid. I panicked and rang for a nurse. They apologized for not informing me that one of the chemo meds, 5-FU, caused this effect. I could taste the chemo as it was being administered and they gave me nausea meds to help with that.

I was told my treatments would be two weeks apart and would have to have blood drawn every Thursday to check my white count. I felt pretty decent on the way home and for the next two days. On Saturday evening we went to a basketball game but before it was over, we had to leave due to my anxiety returning. I felt bad for the kids because they were having a good time. I was up and down all night and for the rest of the week. On Thursday, my white count was border line. A nurse called and cautioned me to be careful as I was susceptible to colds, etc. due to the low count.

Eleven days following the treatment, and taking the red 5-FU, my hair began to fall out. When I ran my fingers through my hair, it came out in bits and pieces – I thought, if I don't touch it, it would stay. I could see hair on my clothes and on my pillow in the morning. Even though I had a wig, and I thought I was prepared, I wasn't ready to be bald. I was NOT prepared. On the 14th day towards evening, I went to take my shower while everyone watched TV. While washing I noticed hair all over the tub floor and my body. I froze, it couldn't be. I felt my head and found the shower water had washed my hair away. Oh, Dear Lord, my hair is gone. I am bald. I called Gene to come to the bathroom and give me a mirror, BUT do not open the shower curtain. He asked me why and I told him I needed to see something and that he should leave. He asked if I was okay, and I told him no but I needed to be alone. When I looked into the mirror, I was appalled and couldn't believe what I looked like. A person's head without hair is white, whiter than your face with an outline of where your hair grew. I was devastated and I cried and hit the wall. I thought I wanted to die, but not really. Now I looked like a person with Cancer. I hate that word. It took me a long time to go out of the bathroom with a towel wrapped around my head. I had a hard time telling my family and it took me quite a few days to deal with the situation. Val came over and measured my head to make me several soft turbans out of terry cloth. I wore them all the time, her daughter gave me one of her favorite hats and I wore it a lot, too. I loved my wig because it looked so natural.

One day I came home and there was cut hair in the bathroom trash can. I hoped one of the girls hadn't cut her long hair on her own. They all had beautiful long hair and I didn't want them to have it gone or messed up. There was more hair in the toilet and around the sides which didn't flush. Everyone was at school and I kept finding hair on the carpets. While putting their clean clothes in their closets, the mystery was solved. In their sympathy with me losing my hair the girls had chopped off their Barbie Dolls' hair so I would feel better. I believe this was their way with coping with their own sadness.

The teachers told me that all of them had become so different and more withdrawn with sadness and worry about their mom. Kandy had even fought with some of the kids, including boys. Jackie was having problems but she wouldn't talk to me about them. They were all so helpful and we spent much more time together. I was so thankful for such great kids to have and to love.

I continued chemo treatments every two weeks and I would feel crappy for a week, then as I began to feel better, it was time to go back again. My white count continued to drop and Dr. T. started me on injections of Neupogen to help increase the white cell count. I went weekly to the emergency room to get those injections. They really hurt and made my bones ache. During these visits I met a couple of girls who became very good friends. I would have to sit in ER for a while after a nurse took my vitals and gave me the injection. Every week I saw one girl and one day I mentioned that I'd bet she got tired of seeing me every week to take my vitals, plus having to sit and visit with me until I could leave. She told me she enjoyed her job and I was always fun to see. She told me she would miss the next week, but would return on the following week. I left and the next week, she was there. Only it wasn't really her. I sat down to have her take my vitals and I asked if she decided not to go this week. The girl asked where she was going? I explained I thought I wouldn't see her for a week and would the following week. Oh, she explained that I must mean Carrisa. I was like "what"! She then explained that she had an identical twin sister. This girl's name was Malissa and they both worked in the ER as CNAs. We both had a good laugh about that. I was seeing both of the girls and thought they were one and the same. And yes, they are identical. No wonder some of our conversations were a bit weird.

Every week it became harder and harder to go, even when three of my friends picked me up to take me to Omaha and give me support. I would call them and say I'm not going any more. They told me to get ready, whether I like it or not, I was going. I always rode in the front seat near the controls as my hot and cold flashes were ridiculous. They didn't come on gradually, it was like Boom and they were there. I could be standing and talking to someone and all of a sudden I would be like a dripping faucet or like a wet rag. Talk about embarrassing.

I had to go through what you call a sandwich treatment. I went from January to June for chemotherapy, then six and a half weeks of radiation, then back for another round of chemo until the end of December. During radiation my mom and dad drove me back and forth every day, Monday through Friday with weekends off. I am so thankful for them and all that they have done for us during my surgeries and all my appointments. I never got too sick during radiation, just tired and burned. I had a large road map on my chest which must not be washed off as they were lines and dots drawn for the radiation to be directed precisely. By this point I am no longer embarrassed to be topless. I would lie on a table while Dr. Z. and his team had to draw and measure for a long time. You lose the sense of modesty and don't think about them looking at you or what are they thinking. Who cares as long as I am alive.

Sisterhood of the Wounded Breast

After several radiation treatments, my skin under my arm became very thin. One day when I was driving home, I reached forward to change the radio station and I felt something warm running down my side. I felt under my shirt and found I was bleeding. My skin tore from reaching forward and stretching it too far. I called Dr. Z. and he gave me some concoction to mix and keep cool in the refrigerator to dab on any time I needed it. It really helped.

During radiation, my hair grew back and I looked like a new baby with brand new baby hair. My kids loved it and always wanted to touch it Once radiation treatments were finished, I was headed back to see Dr. T. to restart those horrid chemo treatments. My thoughts were *No, don't make me*. But I had to so, for the next four and a half months I again had to endure Chemo, nausea, anxiety, numerous meds, hot and cold flashes, low white cell counts, more Neupogen injections, trips to Omaha and Norfolk, plus many calls to the doctors. Again, after two weeks of chemo, I lost my hair. It wasn't fun, but it was a little easier for me this time. Again, my sleep was interrupted with anxiety and I looked terrible. I was determined to beat this evil demon. My family and friend were and are amazing. They stood by me and listened to me cry time and again. I am so blessed with wonderful pastors, from both the Methodist church in Pilger and the Beemer

Mennonite Church who were with us every step of the way.

In October, close to Halloween, my kids were picking out costumes to wear for trick and treating. They thought it would be fun for me to be dressed as Mr. Clean (with the bald head). NOT! What a sense of humor they have!

Thanksgiving and I realized how fortunate and Blessed I am and so Thankful to be alive. God has given me another chance to be with my family to watch them grow, to be able to love them, and to give all they have given me back to them. I reflected on all the pain and suffering that God went through for us and what I thought was the worst time of my life. I thought I was going to die. I thought I wouldn't make it through those treatments, but it was nothing compared to what HE did for us.

At the Methodist Church we have a saying we end with each week which really means a lot to me: God is Good…All the Time…All the Time…God is Good.

December arrived and so did my last treatment! WHO-HOO! I went in for my blood work and Dr. T. said it looked great. He also told me how proud he was of me for hanging in there as he knows it wasn't easy. It felt good knowing this was the last of that yucky tasting chemo. I couldn't wait for my hair to grow back. I had a doctor appointment in two weeks and then they would see how often after that. All the nurses were so excited that I was done. I had to keep my port in for close to a year in case any problems occurred. There were no problems and I went back into surgery to have the port removed. When Dr. R. took it out, he let me see it. I couldn't believe how long the tubing was that is placed down towards your main arteries to run the chemo into your system. No wonder I had been so sick.

Looking back now, I am so thankful for the drug, that I hated so much, that saved my life. My hair started to come back in and at first it was just a layer of real soft, downy, and silky hair. Later, it turned into really thick layers of curly hair that made me look like a boy. My kids laughed because they thought I looked just like one of their classmates who had hair like mine. When it grew longer, it had such tight curls that it was hard to do anything with it. The length was actually past my shoulders, but the curls pulled it so tight that they bounced above my shoulders. The color seemed to be darker that it was originally. I love it. I love having hair and I thank God. I finally had to cut it to be able to manage it and now it is so much easier to handle.

I had to go to the doctor every two weeks for several months, then once every month for a year. I moved to once every three months, then once every six months, and I finally graduated to once a year. I continue on the yearly schedule and go every

December for lab work. I still hate blood work as I am a "hard stick" and they sometimes have to call in their "life-flight" to do the draw with what they call "butterfly needles" due to my small and hard to find veins. They can only use my left arm for the draw since my cancer and surgery was on my right side. I then head to the x-ray department where they do a chest x-ray and follow-up with my doctor appointment.

As I am writing this and looking back on this challenge, I am so thankful for my life. WE have had family ups and downs like all other families. There were times when I felt so helpless during this that I wanted to give up. But with the great God that I have in my life and the faith that my parents instilled in me, I was taught to live and trust. With the awesome family and friends I have, I knew I couldn't just give up. Life is worth living and I wanted to be a part of my families' lives.

(The year of 2013)
Ryan will be 35 this month, Jenny is 32, Kandy is 28 and Jackie is 26. I now have a granddaughter, Alyssa, who is 11 and is one love in my life. She is Jenny's daughter and I am so blessed. In December I will have 19 years of remission (and I still hate that word).

I am now a Registered Nurse and I work the 11-7 night shift at Norfolk Regional Center in

Norfolk, NE. It will be 15 years this year and it all started because of finding a lump in the shower one day.

God is Good…All the Time…All the Time…God is Good.

Chapter Twenty-Three

Mary L. Maas

My first brush with suspicious results of a mammogram took place a number of years ago. When I received the notification of an abnormal reading, I was a bit shaken and returned for a second mammogram. The second test revealed a cluster of micro-calcifications and they were to be watched in future testing.

As the days and months passed by, I think I became complacent about monthly exams, but I did set my annual appointments for a mammogram. There were no aunts, grandmothers, or siblings, who had been diagnosed with breast cancer. I had sisters who had cysts and lumpectomies without malignancy, so I really wasn't overly apprehensive about the yearly visit to the mammography department.

In the late winter of 2009, we got a call from our youngest son telling us that his wife was diagnosed with breast cancer. There was no family history of breast cancer in her relation, either. She had a lumpectomy and had to undergo follow-up treatment of chemotherapy, radiation, and medication.

One year later, my youngest sister was diagnosed with breast cancer. We were all shocked since there was the absence of family breast cancer history in our background. She had a lumpectomy and radiation treatments, along with a preventative medication for five years. The dreaded enemy, Cancer, was marching ever closer amongst our loved ones.

When I retired in 2005, my husband and I began spending winters in Green Valley, AZ. I had conscientiously kept my mammogram appointments before we left Nebraska. But following my exam in 2010, I received another letter to inform me again of questionable areas found. The letter stated they were possibly benign micro-calcifications, but I was to make an appointment for a follow-up test in six months. I wasn't worried at the time and put a note on the calendar to call my doctor to make the appointment in the spring, upon our return to Nebraska.

June, 2011, arrived along with my annual trek to the clinic. Again, the results were abnormal and an appointment was scheduled for the fall, before we left for AZ for the winter. The summer days whizzed by with our 50th Wedding anniversary celebration and a publisher's release of my second pictorial history book. My thoughts and days were consumed with the rush of book signing events and sales opportunities scheduled. All of this busyness kept me from thinking about the portents of that letter.

We were to leave for AZ the first of November, which was a bit earlier than the six month waiting period my insurance required. My doctor made it possible to get tested a few days ahead of time.

This time, the results were not simply considered suspicious, but the radiologist came in to tell me I needed a biopsy. My stereotactic needle biopsy was scheduled for 11-01-11. The roots of fear started to grow and twist in my gut, spreading out from there to fill my head with every scenario imaginable. All the "what if's" assaulted me. The results were positive - CANCER. The utterance of that word alone is enough to instill a growing degree of panic. I knew my life would never be the same.

My husband and I had a conference with my surgeon and we were told that I could have a lumpectomy with follow-up treatments or a mastectomy with not having follow-up with chemotherapy and / or radiation, depending on the results of the surgery. He advised a lumpectomy if I had a treatment center nearby.

We were told that he would excise the problem area and if the margins were not clear, he would go back in and take more tissue until the margins tested clear.

Sisterhood of the Wounded Breast

The date for the surgery was scheduled for 11-11-11. Veterans Day, the annual day for the remembrance and recognition of veterans, especially those who had served during wars and conflicts. I thought after the surgery, I, too, would be fighting to become a veteran of my private war with cancer.

The beginning of my battle was to face my family with the diagnosis. I had a husband who was with me every moment, and walked through every difficult step by my side. I was so fortunate and blessed to have our daughter-in-law, who lived nearby and was so willing to talk about what she had experienced two years earlier with her breast cancer. She talked me through some issues that I might have to face. Many phone calls passed between me and my youngest sister who was going through her time of treatments, reconstruction and other difficulties.

I had wonderful support from my immediate family plus many friends and my church family. My name was added to the prayer list at my home church and at our community churches. That is one of the many blessings of living in a small rural town where everyone knows everyone else and they are there to help in good times and bad. My own prayer petitions for healing and strength were numerous and unending. My faith was firmly rooted in my heart, but my head kept throwing out questions for which I didn't have any answers.

It seemed to ease some of my anxiety to understand what others had already gone through, including my youngest sister's ongoing treatments and results from her breast cancer surgery. However, on the day of surgery, I found myself filled with unbridled apprehension about what I would find when I woke up. I have never come out of anesthesia very well after any of my surgeries and knowing that just added to my worries.

My lumpectomy was done in the outpatient surgery department. Curt stayed with me in the preparation phase and until they took me down to surgery. His face was the first thing I remembered when I came out of my rocky recovery from the anesthesia. He told me the doctor said the cancerous spot was removed and it hadn't spread into any of the surrounding tissue or lymph nodes. The first skirmish of my war was over.

I had an appointment to see my surgeon one week later. If all went well, we would be headed for Arizona right after the appointment and I could make arrangements for my radiation treatments in Green Valley, AZ, our winter home.

The time between my mammogram and the date of surgery was filled with sleepless nights, many tears, and prayers. I wanted to reverse the clock to return to my normal life filled with happy days and plans for a long, long future ahead. I was afraid, despite the surgeon's confidence that it would be taken care of with a lumpectomy and possibly some radiation sessions.

I thanked my Lord for all the support from my family and friends. I thought this was just one more challenge for me to face as I traveled the road of life. This was a bump in the road, not a mountain that I couldn't climb. I considered it a blessing that the surgery was successful and that I had been diagnosed early, before the malignancy got a chance to spread out of the duct.

I am almost four years out from the biopsy and diagnosis of DCIS, Stage 1. I went through surgery and 36 radiation sessions without any complications. I am on a five year regimen of Tamoxifen, which has given me a few irritating side effects, like the return of my long ago and forgotten hot flashes, aching joints, dry eyes, some stubborn weight issues, and daily fatigue. These are more of a nuisance than something that I can't deal with.

I now have a different outlook on life. The little things which seemed so important are not so much now. The aggravations or disappointments that crop up are something to get through with the mantra "This, too, shall pass" is helpful.

I have learned to change what I can and leave the rest in God's hands. The only things that matter are my faith, my husband, my family and my friends. I look at each day as a new beginning, a new venture, to be faced with optimism and the knowledge that I can face whatever is waiting on the other side of the long hill ahead.

One day at a time, take one day at a time, and wake up each morning with a prayer of thanks on my lips and joy in my heart. There is a better and brighter life after cancer for me.

www.ingramcontent.com/pod-product-compliance
Lightning Source LLC
Chambersburg PA
CBHW051902170526
45168CB00001B/205